ALFRED AYOKUNLE

High Achiever

Unlocking The 9 Principles That Transform Your Health, Leadership, and Business

First edition

ISBN: 9798577641382

This book was professionally typeset on Reedsy.
Find out more at reedsy.com

Contents

Why This Book Was Written

It turns out that a lot of people don't know what to do health-wise, how their social circle affects them, and how to become a successful being. I began the journey of writing this book with the hope of showing you a better path to attaining leadership and a healthy lifestyle that ultimately produces success. This book is going to communicate what it takes to be a leader, the characters or traits all great leaders have, and how to control and take advantage of your emotions. After reading this book, you will be able to immediately implement in your life the time tested principles that all high achievers use that produces measurable and sustainable results. Use these principles to your advantage, and you could truly revolutionize your life.

Health and Emotions

This book was written at the time of an ongoing COVID-19 pandemic. There are confusions and disorder around the world. Folks are scared of not having enough money to feed families. Millions of jobs are lost. Everyone is on a tantrum train. Anger is being let loose. At this critical time, the only way to regain one's sanity and become productive is to understand how the brain creates emotions, and how to control those emotions, so that you can live like a high achiever, and not spiral into debt and emotional illness. All successful people are known to have excellent emotional stability, for example, Tony Robbins. Although this book was written in a pandemic period, its teachings can be applied even after the pandemic. People with good emotional health are aware of their feelings, thoughts, behaviours, and are better able to live a good life. However, individuals who aren't able to recognize and manage their emotions would live a struggling life. These uncontrolled emotions will lead to an intense feeling of anxiety, stress, depression, or loneliness.

Leadership and Business

Leadership is vital to have to manage and drive people to work for a common goal to achieve success. A leader is a person who can motivate and influence employees to come together and work effectively and efficiently to achieve a goal. Leadership plays a vital role in the success and progress of any business or group. In the absence of effective leadership, no company or group can work efficiently; in other words, poor results. To become an effective leader, you must be able to:

- Initiate action
- Provide motivation that creates the urge to act
- Create confidence in your team
- Guide your team on how to perform their work
- Instigate change and provide a pleasant working environment

This book is not merely for business leaders or health enthusiast; it's for everyone who has the interest in becoming the ideal parent or employer that understands and foster the emotional and personal needs of a child or employee to allows for successful work life.

It is for anyone who wants to harness the power of the principles all successful professional uses—from having total control of your emotions to developing a leadership skill—that ensures greater work effectiveness and efficiency.

What You Are Going To Learn

The structure of this book is laid out in nine principles:

Principle One

In this principle, you will learn:

1. How anger destroys your social and professional life
2. Strategies to alleviate negative moods
3. How your emotions are created in your brain
4. How fear helped us survive for millions of years
5. The detrimental effect of stress
6. Why CEO's use laughter to build successful companies

Principle Two

In this principle, you will learn:

1. Why you shouldn't please people
2. The reasons for depression and loneliness
3. How to overcome low self-esteem
4. Why self-confidence is collective in successful people
5. How to compare yourself with the right people
6. How negative self-talk affects your social life
7. How your environment influences your behaviours
8. Why peer pressure isn't the fault of your peers

Principle Three

In this principle, you will learn:

1. How gratitude helps you live a happier life
2. How meanings to events affect your moods
3. What importance are your family and friends
4. Why we remember bad experiences more than the good
5. Why a man who lost his wife became relaxed.

Principle Four

In this principle, you will learn:

1. Why self-improvement is necessary for you
2. How books evolved from cave drawings
3. How reading books reduces depression
4. Why seminar is the future
5. How the food you eat is stored and used as energy in the body
6. Why too much food energy is a problem
7. What kinds of food should be included in your diet
8. Why physical activity increases longevity

Principle Five

In this principle, you will learn:

1. Why our ancestors socialized with others
2. How people affect the growth of children
3. Why companies value teamwork
4. How your environment determine your future
5. Tips from executives on how to deal with negative people

Principle Six

In this principle, you will learn:

1. How Steve Jobs, Bill Gate, and Walt Disney became successful with the help of others
2. The 4Cs all successful companies and groups utilize
3. Why Yahoo lost over $40 billion
4. How to mitigate the effect of a blind spot in leadership and business
5. Why Bill Gates, Richard Branson, and Oprah Winfrey have mentors
6. What to look for when choosing a mentor

Principle Seven

In this principle, you will learn:

1. How focus improves your productivity
2. How habits are formed
3. Why habits are essential for success
4. What habits successful individuals have in common
5. Why goal setting lessened Multiple Sclerosis
6. The effects of goal setting in students
7. Why overthinking a step before taking action causes more harm than good
8. Why rest improve productivity

Principle Eight

In this principle, you will learn:

1. The five laws of success
2. Why being responsible is essential for leadership.
3. Signs common to irresponsible people

4. Why success takes time to realize
5. How to leverage the power of time
6. How J.K. Rowlings turned failure into a billion-dollar success
7. Why failure is inevitable and necessary for success
8. Why hard work is so important (perhaps, more than talent)
9. When is the proper time to quit a job or a relationship?
10. How loss aversion and sunk cost fallacy affects your decisions

Principle Nine

In this principle, you will learn:

1. How grit made Stephen Hawking lived longer
2. The equation for high achievement
3. The importance of I.Q. in business
4. Why I.Q. is valued more than E.Q. in a workplace
5. How delayed gratification increase your chance of success
6. Why delayed gratification is hard

This book isn't written just to entertain you (as you will soon experience), but its primary goal is to help you get practical and valuable results. And to get results, you have to put in the work. With that said, let the journey begin.

I

Part One

HEALTH and EMOTIONS

1

Principle #1: Own Your Emotions

One thing you can't hide is when you're crippled inside. — John Lennon.

Emotion is one of the most basic driving force of every human and animal, as well. The way you think, respond, handle a crisis, and show affection to others is largely influenced by your emotions. Emotions make us do things, as the name suggests (remove the first letter from the word). It influences our behaviours—how we laugh, the way we collaborate amongst employees, and how we experience happiness amongst ourselves. Recently, psychologists and researchers have broadly recognized emotional management (or emotional intelligence), which is the ability to understand and control one's emotions (and sometimes others) as an essential skill to achieving happiness, better relationships with others, and success in an organization.

Several studies indicate that up to ninety percent of the decisions we make are based on emotions. In this chapter, we would discuss the following: how to control anger so as not to affect our health and productivity when working, what is the science behind fear, how to manage anxiety to take more actions, the consequences of stress in our health and productivity, the importance of meditation and how it can help boost happiness, how laughter can help build meaningful relationships and improve happiness.

Anger

Anger management is a crucial tool when dealing with a real-life situation (especially when you're surrounded by people whose aim is to piss you off). In our modern world, filled with people in constant hurry to get to work early (with deadlines to meet), or in tattered relationships, or stressed from the incessant studies and homework given to them at school, it is quite easy to find a person or two who would lash their anger and frustration at you and others.

Anger, in many ways, can cause a lot of problems in a person. It can influence sickness, reduce workplace effectiveness, destroy relationships between couples, parents and children, boss and employees, and between employees themselves.

Lulu, a friend, explained to me how anger destroyed the relationship she had with her dad. "I didn't always hate or get annoyed with my dad," she said, "in fact, I had an O.K relationship with him. But everything came to an end on a depressing Friday afternoon." Then Lulu began her childhood story.

I grew up in Nairobi, Kenya, which is a beautiful city, Lulu narrated. When I was young, my mother, Nia, and I worked together in her shop to sell clothing materials in a small town that contained a few thousands of people. Before my parents had money to send me to school, my mom and I would go to the shop, six days a week, twelve hours each, buying and selling clothing materials. At that time, my mother was the only trader selling clothing materials in the town, so she became quite successful within a short period.

My mom and I had (and still have) a great relationship together. After closing the shop for the day, she usually bought me drinks and roadside snacks when going back home. She was also quite patient with me when I indulged in silly activities like dirtying my clothes when playing with my friends, disturbing the neighbourhood with my squeaky screams and noises. I always loved listening to her and responding to her errands because, at the end of each errand, I would usually get candy and a big "thank you" hug, which I love.

"My father, Obama (not what you are thinking)," Lulu chuckled, "on the other hand, is a hard-working man, and a disciplinarian. He works at a steel manufacturing company. My father is, no doubt, an intelligent and handsome man, but what I dislike about him is his lack of patience with the people that associate with him, which I would guess is the reason why he comes home alone from work, even when our close neighbour works with him in the same plant. A year after, my parents got enough money to send me to school (which I desperately needed). The school was the biggest in the town with a lot of synergistic bright colours and beautiful drawings on the inside and outside walls of the school. This was the school every child wanted to be in. The school had the best uniforms that fit well on every student and made every normal kid look handsome or pretty.

I made friends during the first day of class, I could recall. Although I couldn't read well (that was because I had not gone to school prior), my mom and the teachers were generous to help me become a better reader through extra lessons after class. On a warm Friday morning, all students went to the field to prepare themselves for sport. I always loved sports (running mostly). I was in the running team, set to run a relay race that day. Placed to run the last lap of the race, I got intense pressure from within my gut to finish first because I considered myself competitive. I was in the second position when I received the baton from my partner, with the first-position runner about 2 meters ahead of me.

As I tried catching up with the student, my legs failed me (they crossed each other), which caused my fall and lost the race to the first position. While on the floor, on the dusty track, I cried and yelled in pain, because I got seriously injured. Although the wound wasn't deep, the pain was excruciating, especially for a young girl like me. I was immediately taken off the track and attended to. The teacher cleaned and dressed my wounds, and I took glucose so I won't cry further.

In need of assistance, two of my friends followed me home that afternoon—one of them assisted me with carrying my bag. When I got home, I pulled a key out of my bag and opened the door—my parents weren't at home. My friends and I got to my room where I changed clothes and unpack my bags. Suddenly, I heard the door open forcibly. I silently got out of my room, trying to peek who had come into the house ferociously. To my surprise, it was my dad. I thought to myself, *Why is he home so early?* After he came in and sat on the couch, he yelled my name—I guess he noticed my presence because of the sandal I left outside.

I leapt towards him and noticed his frowned face, which looked like he got into a fight. Although he was angry, it wasn't a new thing, but this was different.

"Yes dad," I responded with a shaky voice.

"Prepare me a meal now," he ordered with vex.

I tried preparing the meal as fast I could, but I just couldn't (my injuries wouldn't allow that). Being the eldest child of two children (now, three), I had to do some, perhaps, most of the house duties.

As time passed, he became angrier, waiting for his food to be served. But again, because of my injuries (which he didn't care about), I wasn't able to prepare the food as fast as he wanted. When the food got ready, I served and placed the meal on the dining table, where he was waiting impatiently. Immediately I placed the food on the dining table, I received a massive slap on my face that made my left eye blurry for about three minutes.

"Why are you just bringing the meal?!," he shouted. By this time, I could feel the heat of anger exude out of him as his face begins to steam. "Can't you see (I couldn't see) that I have been waiting for the meal for over an hour?"

That day, I felt hatred towards him and was unfortunate to be injured. I expressed my pain to my father by crying profusely (that was the best I could do). The next day, Saturday, I reported the event to my mom. She became angry instantly. She hurriedly went to meet him where he sat. I heard noises and bangs, I got scared he was going to beat my mom (he didn't), but my mom got so riled up that she almost left the house packing with me along—thanks to the neighbours and family members that convinced her.

"Today," Lulu says in an upbeat tone, "much grown with my own happy family, I have chosen not to speak with my dad because he hasn't changed and he hasn't given me the respect I deserve, albeit I have forgiven him."

Lots of parents out in the world scream, shout and yell at their kid, but the fact is that it accomplishes little to nothing in changing their behaviours. It creates a corrupt relationship between parent and children. It builds fences that separate the children from the patents.

Lulu had a good relationship with her mom because of the love and appreciation her mom expressed to her daily. On the contrary, Lulu's relationship with her dad became worse because of his lack of patience and misunderstanding toward her and her mother.

Did I mention why Lulu's dad came home early that Friday afternoon? He got fired at work when he involved himself in a fistfight with his work colleague for the fourth time (different colleagues, though). Because of his anger, Lulu's dad almost ruined his relationship with his wife and damaged the relationship he had with his daughter and workmates.

Being angry also affects your health in many ways. According to an article published by CNN, shows that people who experienced severe anger outbursts were more at risk for cardiovascular events in the two hours following the outbursts compared to those who remained calm.

Ways to control your anger

Anger management is a valuable tool that can improve your health and improve relationships so that you don't do anything you would later regret. However, anger can quickly become an issue if it leads to outbursts, altercations, or lack of empathy.

1. *Stop talking.* When you're tensed and hot faced, you may feel the urge to let every steamed word out, but you're most likely to say more than you intend to, which could cause more harm than good. When faced with this situation, take a pause and stop. Take a few moments to gather your thoughts before saying anything. When you do this, you would be able to choose your words to diffuse and resolve the situation carefully.

2. *Take a breather.* In the heat of the moment, your breathing becomes shallower and speeds up rapidly. Relaxation skills such as deep breathing exercises, repeating mantras—words, and phrases such as, *I am calm,*

I am relaxed, are good examples to help you become calm and refocus on your environment. When angry, count to ten before you speak; if very angry, count to one hundred. This would reduce the speed of your breathing to normal.

3. *Relax your muscles.* Physical activities such as stretching, running, walking, and meditation (which we would talk about later in this chapter) can help reduce the frustrations, anger, and stress that we might get from the environment or people.

4. *Take time out.* Take a break from your work and from the noise of the cities and also from social media. Go for a hike (maybe with a friend), experience nature filled with its quietness, and surrounding clean air. You may even find this time alone, away from others, so helpful that perhaps, you'd schedule it into your daily routine.

5. *Practice gratitude.* When faced with the heat of the moment, it can be essential to focus on the good stuff you have right here and now. Realizing how fortunate and blessed you are—sight, health, and family—can decrease the anger.

6. *Laugh.* It is not possible to laugh and be angry at the same time. Laughter can be beneficial in improving health, reducing facial wrinkles, improving productivity among people. Watching cat videos, scrolling memes, or watching stand-up comedy is a great way, among others, to turn your anger into laughter.

If there's nothing you can do about the situation, then there's no reason to be angry because it won't make the situation any better. And if there's something you can do about it, then do it, rather than being upset. Anger is a choice, not an involuntary act or decision.

Fear

Inaction breeds doubt and fear. Action breeds confidence and courage.
— *Dale Carnegie.*

Some people live and thrive on fear-inducing activities—extreme sports, public speaking, sky jumping. These kinds of people are adrenaline seekers; they run into dangerous situations without giving it a second thought. In contrast, most of us have an adverse reaction to the feeling of fear—fear of public speaking, fear of death, heights, ghosts, being in control, fear of missing out (FOMO). Allow me to illustrate a scene:

It's night outside, and you're home alone. You just finished watching a zombie movie that brought you chills. You go to your room trying to prepare your clothes for tomorrow's activity, but, suddenly, you hear the doorbell ring. You freeze; your muscle tightens; your heart races. *This is it*, you thought. You remember this is precisely what happened in the zombie movie you watched recently, where a teenage boy heard a door knock and tried to open the door, hoping that it was a rescue team, but he was wrong—it was a zombie who came in and ate him off.

For your safety, you pick up a base bat, thinking a zombie might be behind the door. You think to yourself, *Do zombies ring bells?* But you don't care—you are too frightened. *It could be a zombie*, you tell yourself. Just as you get close to the door, you yell, *Who is behind the door?!* But it turns out to be a friend who had called you four hours ago to remind you of his arrival.

You've probably experienced the scene mentioned above (if you're a zombie fan). Fears set us on edge; there is compares with it. But here are the important questions that you need answers to: Why do we feel fear? What adverse effect does it have on your health? How does it hinder your progress in life? And how can you gain control in a fearful event?

The Psychology of Fear

Fear is caused by a surge of a chemical reaction from the amygdala in the brain that spreads through the body to respond to a fight-or-flight stimulus that causes fast breathing, racing heartbeat, strengthened muscles, opened skin pores to allow for sweat, among other things. The stimulus could be a fast car moving towards you, depression, a knife at the throat, your boss, a ghost, or even zombies. Fear alerts us to the presence of danger or threat, whether the threat is a physical or psychological stimulus.

However, fear is also a beneficial thing to have. It contributes significantly to the existence of the "Homo" genus. It is a natural phenomenon that has helped our primitive ancestors in many ways. During the course of evolution, fear has been a vital emotion that helped creatures increase their chance of surviving perilous situations. Because this trait has been beneficial to our survival, it has then been passed from every creature's prehistoric ancestors down to their offspring. Think about it; the only reason you couldn't jump from a twelve-story building or a helicopter without a parachute is fear (fear of height or death).

How Fear Affects You at Work

I can't add up how many times fear has stopped Ciara from taking a big leap in her career.

Ciara is a graphic designer that works for a photo-editing enterprise. Whenever we meet, most of the time, the conversation would involve her job—her paycheck in particular. She works just as much as her male co-workers, but she complains of being paid less than the males. When I asked her what she thinks the reason is, she said, "gender pay gap."

But is that true?

There's no denying that women in workplaces have usually been paid less than men, and women cannot move up into higher paid positions as quickly as men.

The Bureau of Labor Statistics reported that, in 2013, female full-time workers had median weekly earnings of $709, compared to men's median weekly earnings of $860. But when I asked if she had negotiated on her salary, she replied, *No*.

According to economic research and survey conducted by Glassdoor, in March 2016, only ten percent of employees reported negotiating their salary and getting more money at their most recent job, with men slightly higher than women doing so. In the US, close to three in five (fifty-nine percent) of employees accepted the salary they were offered at their job without negotiating.

Ciara didn't consider herself less experienced or less superior than the men, but she allowed fear to stop her from getting the right amount of salary she was worth. Fear of confronting the interviewer, fear of losing the job, or asking friends and family to help scout new jobs held her back. But there is good news. In 2019, seventeen percent of full- or part-time employees were reported to have negotiated their salary and got more money.

Ways to overcome fear

1. *Educate yourself.* There is a saying, "What we don't understand, we fear." Most of the time, we are afraid of the unknown; we tend to make a significant decision based on little information—we judge people too quickly; we buy materials we don't know much about. Educating yourself with the right information would help you better examine the situation based on facts rather than speculations.

2. *Embrace it.* Like our primitive ancestors, fear stops us from putting our hands on hot metal, surfing lava, or facing lions. Fear keeps us alive and safe. Fear is a survival mechanism that helps us become more aware of our surroundings. So, embrace fear and let it inform your action, but not control them.

3. *Have a positive attitude.* Having negative self-talk can incite fear in you. Separate yourself from negative information that can bring you to fear—a major one is the media. Most of the information that we take in from the news and social media incites fear in us so that we can focus more or take action right now. Surrounding yourself with positive energy people, along with meditation, will help boost your self-confidence, and also improve your breathing and heart rate.

4. *Get help.* Lack of information is a significant influence to cause fear, but there's no way we can know everything just by ourselves. Having mentors, teachers, family, and support groups who are more experienced and knowledgeable will help you grow to become who you desire.

As Judy Blume once said, "Each of us must confront our own fears, must come face to face with them. How we handle our fears will determine where we go with the rest of our lives. To experience adventure or to be limited by the fear of it."

Stress

You are held up in traffic, going to an important meeting that you can't afford to miss. Your plan didn't work out the way you wanted it. You begin to feel stressed as the hypothalamus in your brain tells the adrenal glands to release the stress hormones—cortisol and adrenaline. The rush of cortisol in the bloodstream starts off the fight-or-flight response which makes you more worried and less stable. These hormones cause your heartbeat to rise, increase blood pressure, speeds up metabolism, and energize the muscles.

Stress is a natural psychological and physical response to the situation in life that triggers the fight-or-flight response: war, economic depression, or death of loved ones. However, a perpetual reaction to small or large stressful situations in your life experience, without a proper way to handle the physical and emotional imbalance, can take a toll on your health and well-being. Some of the symptoms of stress on health that could be fatal include: insomnia, low sex drive, weakened immune system, high blood sugar, fertility problems, and heart attack. As the perceived fear diminishes or no longer persist, the hypothalamus would inform all systems to stop the production of cortisol and adrenaline as it goes back to normal.

Stress is normal to have. But when it becomes chronic, it then becomes an issue. Studies showed that chronic stress could result in excessive alcohol use, drug abuse, eating disorders, mental disorders, and stroke. Feeling stressed could have positive effects on situations in our workplace and relationship. You need a certain amount of stress to perform your best at work. You need to understand the right amount of stress that will provide you with motivation, energy, and grit, in contrast to the ungodly amount of stress that can harm your well-being and relationship.

Some of the everyday stressors you should be aware of and prevent include uncertainty, feeling out of control, high expectations of yourself, having more tasks than you can handle, trying to please people, and negative pressure.

Dealing with Stress

Controlling the level of stress hormones in the body is essential to living a healthy life. Here are ways to reduce the stress level in your body.

1. *Get more sleep.* Having the right amount of sleep (7-8 hours a day) can significantly reduce stress. Make sure to have a warm bath and avoid taking excessive alcohol and caffeine during the evening before going to bed. You can also play a piece of slow instrumental music that could allow you to fall asleep quickly.
2. *Manage your time.* Having to manage the kids, working on projects, and spending much time in traffic to an important event can be a lot of work to do, which can raise your stress, which later leads to headaches and anxiety. Allocating your time rightly to your work activities would bring a sense of order in your life.
3. *Talk to someone.* Being stressed and having someone to talk to can be the difference between life and significant illness. As you might have heard, "a problem shared is a problem solved," which means that when we share the issues that cause fear or anxiety with a close relative or a stranger, we get a feeling of security knowing that we have someone to lean on or support us during that period of turmoil.

Laughter

A good laugh makes any interview, or any conversation, so much better.
— *Barbara Walters.*

Laughter is a normal and healthy thing to do. Everyone loves to laugh, and even God laughs ("God, who sits in Heaven, laughs!" – Psalm 2:4). Laughter is a physical reaction in humans that responds to a particular internal and external stimulus; it occurs from hearing, or seeing something jocular, or tickled. Laughter can significantly improve health, relationship with others, and enhances work performance. Research has shown that laughter can relieve your stress and make you more open to others. Laughter, indubitably, is the best medicine.

You might think laughing is unique to humans only, but you would be wrong. In fact, excessive research has shown that dogs, monkeys, and even rats laugh. During the primordial era, laughter was an essential tool in strengthening the relationship between people and caused people to abate anger and forgive sooner. That was important in enhancing the tribe to improve cooperation to increase the survival rate. Humour can help create healthy emotional and physical changes. It connects you to others, boosts moods, enhances the immune system to fight against pathogens, and acts as painkillers.

Laughter is also essential in work. All great leaders have shown to have a sense of humour. A working environment that doesn't allow for laughter or a bit of fun will become an environment lacking zest and pleasure. Humour reduces social distances between people, and it makes leaders less stressful, more approachable, and more supportive. Humour in companies increases morale, productivity, and trust. Research has shown laughter to increase blood flow, reduce muscle tension, and burn calories. One solid minute of laughter can have a similar effect on your body as ten minutes on a treadmill.

In his TED talk, Anthony McCarten said: "Seriousness is dangerous not just for yourself, but also for your society. Seriousness limits us to narrow thinking, rigid ideology, cruelty, and a tunnel vision; whereas, humour obliges us to have an open mind, empathy, and forgiveness." Most successful executives and leaders have a great sense of humour. Humour, in business, fosters creativity, improves teamwork, and increases job satisfaction. Clearance Dero, an American civil rights activist, wrote, "If you lose the power to laugh, you lose the power to think."

Laughter is free and easy to use medicine that I recommended everyone should have daily. When we were children, we would laugh a lot and socialize with people; we would play all day long. Studies have shown that children laugh more than one hundred times a day. But when we became adults, life becomes more serious, chaotic, and debilitating. We work more often (9-to-5 jobs), create a family and care for them, experience the traumas of killings and wars, it quickly became easy to find a reason not to laugh or have fun that allows for the harmful effect of stress on your health and well-being.

Below are some ways to help bring laughter back into your life.

1. *Smile.* Has there been a day you genuinely smiled and felt stressed at the same time? Unlikely. Smiling often, even amid stressful situations, sends a message to your brain that there isn't anything to be worried about, and you are in control. Do you know that trying to fake a smile can reduce your stress level up to half? So smile often. Smiling is also contagious. When you associate yourself with people, practice smiling at them, and notice the effect it has on them. They would tend to respond in a softer tone and become open to you.

2. *Watch stand-up comedies.* When I'm stressed, the first thing I usually do is watch stand-up comedies. A five-minute video is often enough to take me out from a negative emotion into a positive feeling. There are reasons why people listen to stand-up comedians because it abates their stress. So try one, whether you feel stressed or not. You would feel relaxed.

3. *Associate with fun, and playful people.* Having friends that are witty to hang around with can be a great strategy to relieve yourself from external pressure. When you spend time with funny people, comedians, perhaps, their character would rub off on you. Seek out people that like to laugh and make others laugh. Every comedian appreciates a broad audience.

4. *Recall funny events that happened in your life.* When down and alone, take a flashback at past events in your life that you consider ridiculous or childish. Recalling the great times you had with friends and family, rather than the negative, can lighten your heart and bring a smile to your face.

It surprises me how many of our emotional flares can be quenched with something so free and easy to do: deep breathing and laughing. If you're caught up in a negative feeling such as failure, trauma, grief, or loss, remember this: Your stress-inducing thoughts are unimportant. If there's nothing you can do about a situation, then your worries are useless. However, if you have a solution to the case, then stop worrying and just do it.

2

Principle #2: Don't Live A Lie

Wanting to be someone else is a waste of the person you are. —
Marilyn Monroe.

Here's an interesting fact: We spend money we don't have, to buy things we don't need, to impress people we don't even like. Not only is this ideology harmful to our emotional and spiritual health, but it is also wasteful. Focusing on what others expect us to be rather than what we need to be, we lose our truest self. It turns out that when people are lauded for their skin or partner, they become happy for a short period of time, but when mocked, we feel sadness for a longer period. Don't try to please everyone; because that is a battle you can't win.

Here is a nugget: You can't please everyone all of the time, or some people all of the time. Instead, some people some of the time.

We all have goals and dreams we aspire to become, but we sometimes deviate from what we are and who we could be, to the character others want us to be. Now and again, we identify crises when we start questioning our confidence and decisions. Trying to please people or becoming the person we ought not to be has become a significant theme in modern days; we compare ourselves to others, thinking we are not enough, and letting doubt creep into our minds. Based on the things we hear and watch—The Kardashians—we emulate their lives thinking if we can just be like them: do what they do, dress alike, eat alike, then we'll be happy.

Yeah, right.

This kind of mindset paves a way that deviates from your true self. Here is a story to illustrate:

Cleo is a teenager who would willingly but unintentionally deviate from her true self to attract a boy (let's call him, Hamilton). Cleo wakes up every day looking at the mirror before going to school, trying to predict what Hamilton would like and then dress to that taste. "He loves tall girls, so I need to wear a high shoe," she thought in distress. "He loves girls in open dresses. I saw the way he looked at Charlotte; it must be because of her new hairstyle. Her lip gloss was sparkling. I need to do the same." Cleo spends every time trying to be someone she's not. She thought to herself, *I am not good enough. I am not sexy enough. I am too fat. I'm too short. Boys don't like short girls.*

Like Cleo, many of us put on a costume that isn't us. We buy dresses we don't need, and cars to impress people we don't like. We have weddings or birthdays that are so extravagant beyond our savings just to make others jealous. We buy the latest shoes, bags, and hairstyle just because others are doing the same so that we could fit into the culture and become socially accepted.

We watch adverts about a product with sexy models on the screen and compare them to ourselves, telling ourselves that we need to (ad)d more to our lives to be happy. Fortunately, that's not true. There is no need to pretend and be someone else. A large proportion of individuals (especially Gen Y and Z) have been affected by social media—the same tool that was meant to bring us closer together (as Zuckerberg said) has caused people to distance themselves from their true selves, and reduce self-esteem.

Here is a yes or no question: Do you think everyone is happy with their life all day? Even the millionaires? Exactly! And no one should try to be perfect either. Social media is inundated with people with happy faces (some plastic faces, as well), and events—people on vacation in an elaborate beach, having a million-dollar cocktail. A lot of photos are filtered, styled, edited, and cropped, making them fake. But nobody shows their darkest times and moments (which I believe happens a lot).

Here is a quick note: Don't compare yourself with people you see on social media or TV. Comparing yourself with fake people is unhealthy. Know what you want and don't try to be someone else to get it. It is incredible how we're not scared about attracting people to someone we are not. Here's the fascinating thing: We chase people because we feel they have something we don't have, or we think life will instantly be better if we have them in our lives. We want someone who will be present, but hound someone who is distracted. We want someone who will be interested in us, but we bother those who have no desire.

Have you ever noticed that the things that are not good for us always attract us more? It's almost like the way sweet and fatty food is more desirable, or the bad guy and bad girl is more attractive. Have you ever pondered about it?

A study shows that rejection stimulates the part of the brain associated with motivation, cravings, and reward. To lay it simply: We do it because we feel rejected, which means a lack of worth in us, and the only way to prove our value is to receive love from that person. This kind of attitude can later cause various mental severe healths. But we would only address two: loneliness and depression.

Loneliness

Everybody will feel lonely at some point in their life; when we have nobody to sit next to at launch, when we move to a new city, or when we don't have anyone to play with. However, being alone and being lonely are two different experiences. A person surrounded by lots of friends can still feel isolated if they feel empty, less valued, or not understood. A child whose parent transfers him to another school can feel lonely even though other students surround him. Loneliness has been generally considered a global health pandemic. Lonely people crave human contact. They want to be in a social group, but their state of mind makes it more difficult to form such connections with others.

People who don't know their worth, or real value, or lack confidence in themselves often tend to chase other things that they believe would bring worth to them—drugs and alcohol. This would only cause more harm than good in the long run, leading to chronic loneliness and isolation. Loneliness tends to harm the mental and physical health that could afterwards lead to excessive drug use and alcohol, depression, antisocial behaviour, and increase stress levels.

According to a BBC Radio 4 survey, sixteen to twenty-four-year-olds are the loneliest age group. Researchers have found that loneliness is just as lethal as smoking fifteen cigarettes per day! Loneliness is twice as deadly as obesity. Startling, right?

Lonely people are more likely to die prematurely than those with healthy social relationships. Because loneliness is more rampant in our society than ever before (thanks to the internet), it is essential to watch for specific cues that portray loneliness. Below are some of the signs to watch out for.

1. *They care a lot about material possessions.* Lonely people try to fill up their social needs with material things. A lonely person would tend to believe, "if I could just have this phone, or dress, or house, I would feel valued by others and happier." Sadly, that never works. A survey of 2,500 people over six years found that loneliness was likely to lead to materialism, but the same is not valid in reverse. While materialism can be linked to loneliness, materialism does not cause loneliness. People who acquire material possessions just for the sheer joy and fun of consumption are less likely to be lonely than those who sought material possessions as a measure of success or a type of happiness medicine.

2. *They love doing stuff alone.* Lonely people tend to isolate themselves from people because of their low self-esteem. Lonely people spend more time on social media, play games more often, or binge-watch shows. A recent study by researchers at the University of Texas at Austin found that the more lonely and depressed you are, the more likely you are to binge-watch. The researchers conducted a survey on 316 participants from age eighteen to twenty-nine on how often they watched TV when they had feelings of loneliness and depression. The result showed that the more

lonely and depressed the study participants were, the more likely they were to binge-watch TV, using this activity to move away from negative feelings and avoid social interactions.

3. *They hang out with other lonely people.* Just like a smile, loneliness is contagious, too. The spread of loneliness was found to be stronger than the spread of perceived social connections, stronger for friends than for family members, and stronger for women than men. According to research published in the Journal of Personality and Social Psychology, you're fifty-two percent more likely to feel lonely if you are directly connected to someone lonely.

The Psychology of Loneliness

Loneliness is not far from anyone. It can affect both men and women, young and old. Money, fame, power, and beauty can't protect you from loneliness because it is part of who you are. It's encoded into your gene.

Loneliness is a bodily function like hunger. Hunger makes you pay attention to your physical needs. Isolation makes you pay attention to your social needs. Your body cares about your social needs because millions of years ago, it significantly determined your ancestors' survival. During the primordial era, the only way humans could get more food and survive the jungle's perilous track is for our ancestors to socialize and work together as a tribe.

Those who were not able to socialize and bond with the tribe were shunned and left to forage alone. This would mean starvation. Forming connections with each other was necessary for our survival, so our brain grew and became evolved to understand what others thought and felt, and to establish and sustain social bonds. To avoid being isolated, your body came up with social pain. This pain is an evolutionary adaptation to rejection. It's an early warning system to ensure you stop the behavior that would isolate you from the tribe. That's why rejection hurts.

This mechanism for keeping us connected worked great for most of our history until we began building a new world for ourselves. We now have social media that keeps us distracted, video games that take away our time of forming a human connection, jobs that keep us busy from building strong relationships. In the US, the mean number of close friends dropped from three in 1985 to two in 2011. These technologies and tools we have created that were meant to bring us closer together separates us further. The rise of loneliness has increased the presence of health problems. Loneliness makes you age quicker, cancer deadlier, weakens the immune system, heart attack, cognitive decline, increases the risk of death by thirty percent.

When loneliness becomes chronic, your brain goes to self-preservation mode. It starts to see danger and hostility everywhere. Loneliness makes you assume the worst about others intention towards you, which could make you more self-centered to protect yourself; this could make you more socially awkward, cold, and unfriendly than you are.

Below are some of the things you should know to alleviate feelings of loneliness.

1. *Loneliness is normal.* Buffett, Branson, Cuban felt and will feel lonely at some point. You can't fight it, but you can control it. When you feel lonely, it is because something has triggered a memory of that feeling, not because you are, in fact, isolated or alone. Ask yourself, *Why do I feel this way? Who am I not reaching out to? Do I really need to buy that?* Figuring out the cause of your feeling of loneliness can be a great way to prevent it from spiralling into chronic loneliness.

2. *Be sociable.* Do something you wouldn't normally do. Write to a friend you haven't spoken to in a while, call a family member, invite a work buddy for a coffee, go to a sports club, or a music concert. Be open and vulnerable to other people's affection. You can reach out to people and offer them help. Get outside of yourself and be available for someone else.

3. *Don't think little of yourself.* Thoughts like, "I am not good enough, I am not popular, I have no friends," should be removed from your mental vocabulary and replace with words like, "I have value, I am confident, I am smart, I am unique and special." This kind of thoughts and words would help lift your spirit and sense of self-worth.

4. *Get professional help.* If you realize your loneliness has morphed into chronic loneliness, and it's eating away your health and mental well-being, and you know you can't handle it alone, please do reach out and get professional help. It is not a sign of weakness, but of courage.

Remember, loneliness is a normal feeling. Most animals get what they need from their physical surroundings; we get what we need from each other. Be sociable.

Depression

A survey published by the Centers for Disease Control and Prevention (CDC) showed that during 2013–2016, 8.1 percent of American adults, aged twenty and over, had depression in a given two-week period. Women (10.4 percent) were almost twice as likely as were men (5.5 percent) to have had depression. Depression is a mood disorder that may be described as a feeling of loss, sadness, or lack of social interaction. Year after year, there are more cases of people being depressed. Depression is a severe medical condition that can get worse if not treated quickly or adequately.

Everyone feels sadness, loss, or stress at some point in time, but a persistent feeling of grief and stress can lead to depression. According to the World Health Organization (WHO), depression is the leading cause of disability worldwide and is a significant contributor to the overall global burden.

The symptoms of depression include:

- Changes in appetite.
- Unintentional weight loss or gain.
- Lack of sleep or too much sleep.
- Feeling of worthlessness or guilt.
- Reduced interest or pleasure in activities once enjoyed.

The symptoms of depression may be experienced differently among men, women, and children.

In Men

Men are less likely to be depressed than women, and the symptoms can vary. When faced with feelings of sadness and loss, men are more likely to drink alcohol in excess, express anger, and feel irritated. Here are other symptoms of depression a male may have:

- Express abusive behaviors.
- Feeling hopeless and empty.
- Unable to meet work responsibility.
- Avoiding social interactions.
- Having difficulty concentrating.

In Women

In the US, about 15 million people experience depression each year, and majorities are women. Only about one-third get the help they need. Up to one in four women is likely to have an episode of severe depression at some point in life. Here are some symptoms of depression that tend to be prevalent in female:

- Suicidal thoughts.
- Fatigue.
- Restlessness or excessive crying.
- Having difficulty making decisions.
- Loss of pleasure or interest in activities (including sex or relationship).

In Children and Adolescent

According to a report published by the CDC, 3.2 percent of children aged three to seventeen years (approximately 1.9 million) have diagnosed with depression. Having another disorder is most common in children with depression: about three in four children aged three to seventeen years with depression also have anxiety (73.8 percent), and almost one in two have behavior problems (47.2 percent). Children affected with depression typically have difficulty learning and handling their emotions. Other symptoms of depressed children may include:

- Trouble concentrating on schoolwork.
- Feeling worthless.
- Excessive crying.
- Reduction in energy.

Below are some of the things you can do to alleviate the symptoms of depression.

1. *Socialize with people.* Spending time with family and friends could be a great way to eliminate or reduce depression. Try to go out more often. Look at your society and see what you can do to help. The idea is to spend less time focusing on yourself and more on others, which leads to a positive feeling.

2. *Eat healthy.* You are what you eat. Eating the right food could provide the brain with the proper nutrients to mentally and physically develop itself to more excellent health. A low-fat diet, rich in fish (especially Omega-3), and folic acid helps with the mood. Avoid taking alcohol and caffeine. According to a study in the Archives of General Psychiatry, diets rich in nuts, fish, fruits, and veggies are linked to a lower risk of developing depression.

3. *Meditate.* Affirmations like *I am at peace, I am in control, I have all I need, Today is going to be a great day,* helps to create a sense of calm and peace into your day. Meditations have been proven to improve memory and control emotions, helping manage anxiety, stress, and depression. Spend at least ten minutes of your time each day practising meditation.

4. *Don't blame yourself.* A common theme in people that are depressed is that they tend to blame themselves for specific events that occurred, "I should have done this differently," "if I had known, I wouldn't have..," "it's my fault." But these kinds of constant thoughts are not productive to one's health and would only lead to depression. You have to understand and accept that there are certain things you can't change

and focus on the things which are present that you can change.

5. *Have a positive attitude.* Having a positive attitude can never bring you harm. A positive attitude changes everything. Redefining your mental outlook by expecting good things to happen and being optimistic about situations, interactions, and yourself can change your state of mind from a depression to a blissful experience. Attitude is everything, so think positive.

Overcoming Low Self-Esteem

Developing high self-esteem is essential to become a good leader in the workplace, maintaining a happy relationship, and becoming satisfied with oneself. As Alan Cohen said, "To love yourself right now, just as you are, is to give yourself health. Don't wait until you die. If you wait, you die now. If you love, you live now." Having higher self-esteem means loving and developing self-worth. Self-esteem isn't about thinking you're perfect—no one is, nor is it about bragging. It is about knowing what you are good at and not so good at. Self-esteem is about seeing yourself positively and realistically. So if you know you are good at baseball but not basketball and you feel proud of yourself, it means you have good self-esteem. Here is a story of Kelvin Systrom to illustrate the point:

I was born on Dec 30, 1983, in Houston, Massachusetts, to a fortunate family. My father was the vice president in human resources for a department store corporation, and my mother was a marketing executive for many dot-com companies, including Zipcar. Similar to my mother, I was attracted to technologies and computers. By playing computer games, I began creating my levels out of curiosity. If there's one thing I know about myself is this: if I'm obsessed with something, I would completely immerse myself and try to know everything about it. That's who I am. This behaviour allowed me to focus intensely on my schooling, where I was accepted into Stanford University. But for me, the school wasn't my thing—it was boring.

I wanted to do something that could be applied in everyday life. So I majored in management science and engineering. In my free time, I would build programs and games for friends and for fun. I interned at multiple places, my favourite being a podcast sharing startup called ODEO. I learned from various books and people, including the founders of Twitter. I felt alive and was willing to learn more. So I finished my internship, and during my senior years at Stanford, I got a job at Google.

I was their associate product marketing manager—managing Google calendar, G-mail, documents, and other products. At first, I was thrilled to be there, but after two years, I had the desire to do more—I wanted to create something fresh and become an entrepreneur. So I quit my job at Google and spent hours building my app, formally called "Burbn." It was a prototype app that allowed people to check-in and post photos, but it led me to create one of the most widely used apps—Instagram, which was later sold to Facebook for a billion-dollar.

This was the story of Kelvin Systrom, together with Mike Krieger, creators of Instagram. Like Kelvin, people with self-esteem dare to try out new things, even when their dreams may seem blurry or difficult to reach. When they make mistakes, they always believe in themselves and move forward. Here are some of the things you could do to develop self-esteem.

Develop self-confidence in yourself

What do Steve Jobs, Elon Musk, Leonardo Da Vinci, Warren Buffett, and Wright Brother all have in common? They possess self-confidence in their work ethic. Confidence comes from the Latin word "*fidere*," meaning "to trust," therefore, having self-esteem is having to trust one's ability. Not everyone has self-confidence.

People who lack confidence have difficulty speaking up and prioritizing their own needs, wants, and feelings. They always feel sorry, pitiful, and guilty for things they have no control or responsibility for. They don't feel they deserve more or capable of having more; they have constant abusive internal dialogue; they have difficulty making choices. Life is always a struggle for them. But when you grip the helm of self-confidence, life becomes your theatre.

Here is a story of how Howard Schultz, CEO of Starbucks, made a multibillion-dollar company with self-confidence:

I grew up poor in Brooklyn, New York. My family didn't have a lot of money. My mother was a receptionist, and my father was a World War II veteran, working as a diaper delivery driver. They didn't have a college education, but they worked hard for the family, and they loved their work. It was difficult seeing hard-working people struggle for survival. Then I promised myself it wouldn't happen to anyone else. Most people worked their first job at eighteen. My first job was at twelve-years-old.

I sold newspapers and worked in a local café. I wasn't a straight-A student, but I was good at American football. It was a way for me to escape my world and enjoy something I was good at. I always knew I wouldn't become a professional football player, but I did know I wanted to be educated; I worked hard for it and became the first person in my family to graduate. At twenty-six years old, I became vice president in charge of sales for a Swedish houseware company—it's not IKEA.

This was a big deal, but I didn't feel happy or fulfilled until I visited a large shop that placed orders on one of our items: a coffee maker. At the time, the two owners were selling whole coffee beans, teas, spices, and coffee making accessories. I felt their passion for something as simple as coffees. I knew this was where I belonged, and I fell in love with what they had created.

After calling, nagging, and asking them for me to join their team, I became their marketing director. I visited Milan, and what I experienced was a complete difference from the American coffee drinking culture. People sat down and enjoyed their drinks. It was more than a drink; it was a relationship. That was what we needed, I thought. I told the owners of my vision, but they wanted to stay right of their current business of selling bulk items, not individual drinks. I didn't blame them. America, at the time, didn't even know what a latte was.

I decided I would create my own coffee shop, but the challenge was trying to raise $1.6 million in a year. I spoke to 242 people, and 217 said, No—that's 90 percent, No. They told me it wouldn't work, that it wasn't worth the money. It was challenging, and I was discouraged, but I was after my dreams to become a reality. I didn't get my $1.6 million, but it was enough to open my first shop. We were making about half a million dollars annual sales. I was a step closer to my goal, but something was still missing. Remember the store I had to be part of? Soon after, the owner decided to sell their business, so I bought their six stores for $3.8 million and combined my stores with their six, and I became the CEO of Starbucks Coffee.

Without the confidence and belief that Schultz had in himself, Starbucks wouldn't have existed. Without the confidence the Wright brothers had in their vision, there wouldn't have been commercial planes flying over your head. Every innovative product, technology, scientific discoveries, and long relationship are all founded on self-confidence. Here are steps you can take to develop confidence:

1. *Love yourself.* The first step to having confidence is to love yourself. Many people spend their time making other people happy but at the expense of stressing themselves out. If you feel you are always going out to other people's events—birthdays, music concerts, or watching sports, and you feel burned out, here is your solution: say No. Because we want to make everyone happy or appreciate us, we tend to say yes to people's request all the time, which will cause you lots of pain. Remember this: You can't please people all the time. You should always be yourself.

2. *Stop the negative self-talk.* It can be quite easy to have negative thoughts running through your minds on an endless track. Words like, "I am not smart enough, not attractive enough, not good enough," always make you lock yourself down. Develop a positive attitude and speak positive affirmations to yourself each day, such as, *I am powerful, I am smart, I am blessed.* Remember, you are what you think.

3. *Set yourself up to win.* When you wake up each morning, exercise, meditate, set realistic goals you want to achieve before the day ends. When you are faced with a challenge, pause, reassess, and then move on. Surveys have shown that people who are deliberate and set goals tend to

achieve more than those who don't.

Compare yourself to the right people

Comparing ourselves with others is natural, and sometimes, a good thing. Comparison with others could help provide you with the motivation you need to become just as good as the other person, or even better. Here is a story of Jasper that illustrates the point:

It was school period on a fateful Tuesday afternoon; I was having a physics class. During the lecture, the teacher decided to throw a surprise quiz.

Gasp!

Everyone was shocked, terrified, eyes bouncing around, students mumbling and in dread. But there was a student who wasn't. He was as calm as a snowflake. His face exuded readiness. (Let's refer to him as John).

I, in particular, was shocked. I thought to myself, "Has he read the material, or didn't he hear what the teacher just said?"

Despite our cries, the teacher began with the quiz. As far as I can remember, only a few of us answered the question correctly, but the majority was answered correctly by the calm, well-prepared student.

After class ended, I went to meet John and asked how he got to answer most of the questions correctly. Fortunately for me, he was generous and kind enough to tell me how he studied and what he does each day after school ended.

When I tried implementing his study plan, it felt arduous, and I definitely wanted to quit. But when I felt low on brain juice, I would tell myself, "Why can't I complete this study? If John can complete the study each day, why can't I? He doesn't have two brains." These words pushed me to develop the habit of reading. Two weeks later, we had another quiz. This time, I was a bit calm, more prepared, and ready. After the quiz ended, John and I got the two highest points.

Stories like this happen every day in our society. We compare ourselves to co-workers, our boss, our spouse, colleagues, and sometimes, children (not weird at all). But when we compare ourselves to people with a much higher level of ability or work ethic, it can cause burnout and make us unhappy with ourselves, even when we have enough.

For example, an amateur in tennis (like me), should not practice or compare himself or herself with a professional like Serena Williams. Comparing or competing with a person that's way ahead of you in tennis, or other things for that matter, can make the game boring for both participants, make you feel like a loser, and could make you not want to try anymore. If I were to play a tennis match with Serena Williams, there are chances that I would not get a single point. And that for me would make the game less motivating and boring for the other participant, also.

So when trying to compare yourself to others, make sure to compare yourself to people that have a slightly higher ability than yours. For instance, if I have a tennis skill level of 1, and am hoping to get to Williams' level of 20, it would be energy-draining to try to compete with her directly and hoping that someday I would reach her level. I would have quit before that could happen. But, say, I was to compete with a person with a skill level of 5, now the chance of me winning or getting points is much visible, which would help boost my motivation to keep on training that would cause growth. Note this: Compare yourself to the right people, with the right ability close to yours. Make sure it builds you rather than demotivate you.

Appreciate what you have

Knowing that you've achieved a lot and have a lot to be thankful for can help boost self-esteem. Many people always complain about what they don't have: I am not tall enough, I don't have the trendiest shoes, I don't have the perfect body; but people do little or never try to appreciate the good things they do have around them—healthy children, supportive family, a functioning body, a purpose in life, excellent health, a house to sleep in, food to eat, and clothes to wear. Before you complain about anything, ask yourself, *Have I been grateful for my health? Have I been grateful for the car I have? Have I been grateful for the food I just ate? Have I been grateful for the life of my children?* Think about that. We live in a very distracting world, where everyone is always on their device in social media, looking at the guys and girls that have the most extravagant houses, cars, or lions. Distracted by the continuous bombardment of advertisements on TVs, billboards, and magazines, we convince ourselves that we don't have enough until we dress a certain kind or have a certain product.

Silence the inner critic

When it seems the world is crashing down on you, or can't escape from your mind, giving yourself a pep talk can do magic. Remind yourself of how awesome, creative, and powerful you are. Sometimes, the only way to silence your inner critic is to drown it with positive words and thought. It's time to stop being your own worst enemy. When you wake up each morning, tell yourself these words:

- Today will be my day.
- I am the best me there is.
- I know that I am a winner.
- I can do it.
- God is always with me.

And while you are about to sleep you can say these words:

- I choose peace.
- Tomorrow is going to be great.
- I am grateful.
- I am blessed.

Having a good night sleep can help calm your mind and bring peace to you. Don't hesitate to have a good sleep, even during the day, if you feel energy drained. It is not a sign of laziness, but wisdom. In a nutshell, when you are going out with a friend or on a date, make sure to think big of yourself. People respect those who believe they are essential. People would judge you based on the way you see yourself. Having self-esteem tells people, "He is smart, intelligent, successful, and dependable. He respects himself, and I respect him, too." Folks will treat you the way you treat yourself. Remember: Your action is the reflection of your thoughts.

Until you begin to focus on the things you have and not the things you don't have, you will never be happy. And as Aristotle said, "happiness depends upon ourselves." Don't let the fewer things you don't have distract you from the many, many things you do have. Happiness and satisfaction are not in the distant future; instead, it is available to us in the present moment.

Survey Your Circle

It was 2014, on a warm Thursday afternoon at the beach. The waves were roaring. Hundreds of people were mingling together with children having fun with the wet sands. Jeremiah and his family came to visit the beach on this very day, as well. Jeremiah is a tall, handsome freshman with black curly hair and a dark-blue eye. His shorts were sky-blue, with an armless top. Anyone could notice his well-shaped body right through his clothing.

After spending some time with his family, a college friend of his came to pick Jeremiah up to attend a friend's party. He excused himself from his family and went along with his friend. On getting there, he could tell from a mile away that the party had already started. On getting out of the car, the first thought that came to his mind was, "This is a Bacchanalia."

When he got in, the atmosphere of the room was loud and disordered along with rising voices and raucous music sounds from all corners of the room. Jeremiah was greeted by lots of friends, and some people he had never met before. Both boys and girls at the party seem to be having fun. There was a lot of grinding, kissing, and other stuff you could think of. The table supported a plethora of booze including Vodka that is poured into disposable cups. Drinks were copious, as well as weeds. Jeremiah wasn't unfamiliar with this kind of party; in fact, he had thrown such a party in the past, however, this was going to be different.

All of the visitors came with a partner or was giving one—that was the theme. Jeremiah, on the other hand, didn't come with one. After several wild screams and erratic dancing, a group of boys decided to exclude themselves from the main party and have their mini party in a separate room—Jeremiah was included. The boys in the group added their girlfriends to join them to spice things up a bit. After settling in, some boys brought out weeds, others brought cracks, methamphetamine, heroin, and other hard drugs. While some brought drinks.

They decided to play a little game that had penalties when someone loses, and the consequence of losing is to consume one or two of the hard drugs or drinks the winner demands of the loser. Before the game commenced, Jeremiah explained to his friends that he wouldn't be able to participate in such an activity. All of his friends were pissed by his remark. They (including the ladies) called him a chicken for trying to chicken out before the game even started.

To clarify, Jeremiah isn't new to drinking and smoking, however, he is nascent to some of the hard drugs brought on the table. They warned him that if he were to chicken out he wouldn't get the girl they had arranged for him to have fun with (the girl was in the room, as well). Jeremiah had a girlfriend, but I guess he wanted to prove that he wasn't a baby, so he decided to stick around. Jeremiah thought it would be foolish of him to lose his friends' respect for him.

But those should have been the last thing he should have feared losing.

After a couple of rounds, Jeremiah lost the game. It was time for him to face the consequences. To redeem himself, he would have to snort a crushed benzodiazepine (also referred to as benzos or French fries on the street). But that wasn't all. He would also have to drink, at least, half a bottle of spirit (sometimes called "shorts"). These types of narcotics (including marijuana, heroin, and fentanyl) raise you high and then drop you low; in Jeremiah's case, it dropped him low to almost beneath the ground. Supposing Jeremiah knew what he was about to do, he would have called an ambulance, prior.

After a few minutes that he had drunk and snorted, his pals cheered and praised him. They handed him the girl and prepared a little room for them to stay. Although he wasn't feeling quite well, everything seemed to be working out fine, up until the process he tried pulling his pants ... and then it happened ... Jeremiah fell and passed out.

An ambulance was radioed immediately and his parents were informed. Jeremiah was brought into the hospital in a coma. His family was terrified. They couldn't fathom how their kid in one minute could be having a good time with them lying in the sands of the beach, and in another minute would lie in a hospital bed, in a coma! The police were involved and interrogated his friends. On the fourth day, in the hospital, he was able to open his eyes and respond to his mother's call.

You might be familiar with this kind of story, however, I think we all know who (or should I say what) the real culprit is ... Peer pressure.

Peer pressure is an immense (but sometimes, subtle) force that wields our choices and behaviours. You will and have experienced the effect of this force at some point. Anyone can testify to that. Before the end of my teenage years, I was a gambler—an addictive gambler. And the only reason for that was because I associated myself with people who were gamblers themselves. A myriad of things influences our decisions in various ways, and if you're not equipped with the right system to combat the subtle forces that compels you to make stupid and dangerous actions, you might end up in a coma, or even worse.

The purpose of writing this section is to help you grasp the impact of the people you accept into your circle and how the setup of your environment can make your life better or worse.

You and People

I'm not in this world to live up to your expectations and you're not in this world to live up to mine. – Bruce Lee

There's no doubt that peer pressure is a real thing and it has become a social issue. Its effect is most prevalent in teenagers—as part of their brain that's responsible for risk assessment, judgment, social, and sexual behaviour control isn't fully developed. The people we hang out with determines who we become and dictate what we do (even in subtle manners). Think about it: haven't you done something(s) that on a normal day you wouldn't see yourself doing, all because your friends also indulge in it. And the interesting part is: they don't have to force you before you begin to do what they do.

If you have lots of friends that love to party, you'll party with them more often than you would normally have if you didn't have such friends. When you continuously accommodate friends that drink alcohol, without any form of pressure from them, you'll likely do the same. And from there, you become an alcoholic.

You might agree that the pressure from our peers is the most important reason for people's irrational actions and behaviours, but I think that's the wrong way to look at it. I would say, the subtle force or pressure that shapes our decisions and behaviours isn't actually from our peers but from ourselves. We do what we do, not because our friends forced us, but because of our desire to feel socially accepted and belong to a certain group. The reason why that gentle and studious girl or boy wants to get laid at such a young age is that they want to feel important and accepted by their friends. Most people would have chosen not to have sex at an early age if not that they want to prove to one person or another that they have the guts to become part of them and to be respected.

I've had conversations with several girls who told me that they had underage sex all because of the pressure from their girlfriends to be regarded as mature. As a teenager (or any person, really), to be assertive, aggressive, athletic, dominant, and hooking up with the opposite sex (or same-sex) is all that's required, especially as a male, to be regarded as a real man or woman by peers. To have sex or to be an alcoholic, as a teenager is almost like an obligation or kind of duty rather than a personal desire. In this century, reputation is all that matters.

A good example of losing oneself for the opinion of others happens within a fraternity. A lot of the frat brothers would say that they wouldn't have gone along with the hazing if they had the choice to quit. But the thing is, they could have stopped if they wanted to and no one would hinder them. I've met people who have quit the fraternity because of the horrendous rituals they have to go through. I believe the main reason why many people fail to leave the frat is that they are afraid of being bullied and mocked by the "brothers." Because of their reputation and how they are going to be judged in college, people continue to lose their lives in the process.

It is this attitude of trying to prove to others and trying to belong to a group that makes us do stupid stuff. The desire to fit in might result in you:

- Snorting, smoking, drinking alcohol, or using other hard drugs.
- Involving in sexual activities.
- Wearing the same brand or style of makeup, or the same form of dressing or hairstyle as your friends.
- Changing the way you talk, or your choice of words.
- Involving in risky or illegal activities.

Jake is a forty-five-year-old accountant. He has been an accountant for over a decade. He has received lots of accolades from his boss several times for his productivity and skill. He is married to a beautiful blue-eye lady, with two children. After spending about six years and a half in his place of work, he formed a very close relationship with three of his coworkers. Occasionally, Jake and his coworkers would go to the bar and have some drinks together and talk about work, and family. This went on for quite some time.

Jake dearly loves his wife and children. He prices them above anything in his life, and his coworkers admire him for that. His coworkers, on the other hand, aren't as committed to their wives and children. Whenever Jake spends time with his three friends, they usually seem joyous and free. At the club, his friends would have drinks and spend time with women on different occasions. Anytime his friends went to meet the pretty women, he would feel left out.

The next day, during a work break, Jake's friends would always talk about the fun they had last night with the ladies. Though Jake's friends consider him a lucky man for having a pretty wife and good children, he interpreted his life as mundane while he interpreted their lifestyle as liberating. So he told his friends about his feelings and they decided to help him. He wants to fit in and feel accepted. They arranged to meet at a special club the next day.

On the first day of the meeting, they hooked him up with a slender, well-figured lady and excused themselves. After several minutes passed, he and the lady went to a room and stayed throughout the night. The next day at work, his face was lit with euphoria from last night's experience. Everyone seemed to be happy about his new adventure. He smiled, joked, and asked his friends to do it again next time. They acquiesced. At this point, Jake could feel the rush of truly being a member of the group.

These events went on for over two months, while Jake was still with his wife. But on one unfortunate day, a friend of Jake's wife caught him and pictured Jake in the action of talking and smooching with another lady. A few weeks later, his wife took the action to divorce him and took the children. That was the beginning of his downfall.

After his divorce and losing his children, he became restless and confided in drinks and women to ease his anguish. His friends felt sorry for him and suggested he should sleep with more women and probably he would find his match.

On one fateful night, the two women he had arranged to sleep with drugged his drink so he would sleep off. While he was asleep, the women robbed him and used his credit card to purchase lots of clothes and accessories online. They utterly wrecked him. The women were savages. All they left for him was his clothes, shoes, and a nearly empty credit card. After being robbed, he became even more restless and unstable, which later cost him his job.

Jake lost everything—his wife, children, wealth, and his sanity—all because he wanted to fit into the tribe. The price we pay to feel loved, valued, and accepted by people that are of no good to us is usually beyond what we can handle. When you don't love yourself and you see yourself as an inferior being to others you feel the pressure to belong and act like others around you.

Jake's story isn't unique, it's what many teens and adult face today. You might say that Jeremiah was forced or pressured to play the game that later put him in a coma, however, if you look deeply, you'll notice that no one forced him to play the game. He could have left if wanted to, but he chose to play on all because he cared more about the opinions of his friends, and less about himself. He wanted respect from his peers at the expense of his life.

As Jeff Moore rightly put it, "Peer pressure is the pressure you put on yourself to fit in." He also said, "You would have no peer pressure if you cared less about the opinions of others." You have to understand that peer pressure is less external and more internal. The choices we make are that which we choose to make—it's a choice. The best way to overcome negative peer pressure is to love yourself more and care less about what others say about you.

You and Environment

Since the day of inception, humans have been inclined to be sensitive to their surroundings to survive. The moment a child is born, his senses kick into gear. He begins to pick on the cues around—scents, touch, light rays, voice. We have an innate awareness of our environment and adjust to the changes being created. When the temperature is low, we put on thick clothes to warm the body. When the noise is unbearable, we move away from the source. When the light rays rushing through the retina become overwhelming, we put on shades to mitigate the rays. When we taste pungent food, we squeeze our faces in disgust and abstain from it. These cues drive our behaviour to act in certain ways or take certain actions all for the benefit of our survival.

Like the way temperature, noise, light, and humidity subtly affect our decisions so does our environment in general. We are the product of our environment. Each of your behaviours stems from the things you have been exposed to from childhood. I want you to look at the things you've been doing from walking, talking, eating, dressing, and dancing; all of these actions have been influenced, at some point, by one or two people. You might think the way you eat is just the same as you've been eating since childhood, but that's not true.

If you look at the way you dress now, I can almost predict with 100 percent accuracy that your style of dressing has changed over time. If I ask why that is so, you might respond, "Well, because, that's just the way I've always been." For most ladies (and guys, as well) their current style of dressing didn't stem from their innate penchant for that style but comes from the models and celebrities they've been exposed to. If you ask the ladies why they use certain brands of products, most will tell you, "Because I've always loved their products. It's smooth, creamy, and it doesn't wear off, blah blah blah." However, if you look deep down and study them, you'll notice that that's false. They do what they do because a celebrity they love is an ambassador for that product. Before then, they've probably seen that same product everywhere in the market but didn't notice it or didn't enjoy using it. But the moment they spot it with a celebrity, they become users and even street ambassadors. That's why you see brands hire celebs to feature in their advertisement because the brands know that even if the majority of people don't like their product, the moment a celeb features in it, it becomes a success.

Such kinds of marketing have become more popular today for anyone who has the money to pay. I once read an article that reported that Paris Hilton, a media personality and businesswoman, during her prime time used to charge anywhere from $500,000 to three-quarters of a million, just to show up at a party or event. Business Insider had an interview with Ryan Schinman, founder of Platinum Rye Entertainment and RBS Celebrity Booking, which connects brands to celebrities and brokers deals for ads; he also helps regular millionaires book entertainers—rock stars, pro athletes, rappers, and the likes to their birthday, weddings, and other events.

In the interview, Schinman said that the cost of hiring a celeb to your event is much lower than what advertisers pay for a commercial shoot. However, he also said, "When you're talking about bands, though, big bands, they are still going to cost you a lot of money. The biggest names in the music business usually go anywhere between $600,000 and $1.5 million, depending on who they are." To get Elton John to sing at your party, it's going to cost around a million dollars! You might be wondering, "Why would anyone pay such an amount of money just to invite a celeb?" One of the reason is: To get prestige and status so that friends and foes would like and respect them, or to make certain people jealous. Whichever their aim is.

Going back to how the environment influences you. The reason why a restaurateur was willing to pay Paris Hilton huge fees just to show up is that they know the moment the public can see a high-profile celebrity at their restaurant, their perception and attitude for that restaurant changes. The moment you spot a celeb that you adore going into a restaurant, even if you've never eaten in that restaurant, you become curious to know why your idol or mentor would dine in such a place. Out of that curiosity, you'll book a table (even if it's expensive). Boom! The marketing stunt worked.

Do you remember Travis Scott McDonald's? The $6 meal that contains a quarter pounder with cheese, bacon, and lettuce, a Sprite, and fries with a barbeque dipping sauce became a success to the point that almost all Mcdonald restaurants were out of fries and other ingredients.

Brands are always on the lookout for the trendiest celebrity and are willing to pay a premium price to get them. When we notice people we admire, we behave in certain ways that tend to model them in an almost precise manner. We want to feel what they feel, eat what they eat, and use what they use, almost in a way to become as ONE.

To wrap this chapter up: The way you eat, smile, dance, walk, and your penchant for other activities isn't as innate as you might have thought but stems from your environment—what you've been exposed to from childhood. Because of the subtle, but huge impact your environment can have on you, it's salient to always meticulously choose what you expose yourself to.

3

Principle #3: Live And Appreciate The Moment

If you concentrate on what you don't have, you will never, ever have enough. — Oprah Winfrey.

Have you ever felt like you are not getting ahead? Like you don't have enough? Or like you don't have anything meaningful going on in your life? These are questions that many will respond yes to, without a second thought. But are those responses really true?

A large number of individuals don't focus on the moment and appreciate what they have around them, no matter how small it might be. We have a lot to be thankful for than we think. Do you know that if you have a family, a house to live in, a proper education, three square meals, a complete body, and a proper smartphone, you're living more comfortably than over seventy percent of the global population?

Are you now convinced that the things you have around, that are so common, are the things you need to be thankful for? A lot of sadness and pain would be eliminated if only we would appreciate the moment. The reason for the perpetual feeling of lowliness and gloom is that we tend to focus less on what we have "here and now", but focus more on what we don't have or what we could get in the distant future.

Rather than attempting a quick-fire list of ways to appreciate the moment more, I have chosen to focus on a select few—gratitude, focus on here and now, and attaching a positive meaning to life—that would expand your horizon on how to interact more with the things you have, and feel happier about it.

Gratitude

Gratitude is the expression of being thankful and the readiness to show appreciation. There is scientific evidence that shows gratitude to be linked with happiness. Gratitude helps people feel positive emotions, improves health, build strong relationships, enjoy a good experience, and make you more productive. Expressing gratitude changes the brain's molecular structure, which keeps the gray matter functioning and makes us healthier and happier. When you show and receive appreciation, the brain releases dopamine (a feel-good chemical) and serotonin, the two crucial neurotransmitters responsible for regulating our emotions, appetite and digestion, memory, and pleasure.

They play a vital role in how good and happy we feel. Humans usually care less for the everyday things they have but should be grateful for, such as:

- the food we eat,
- the bed we slept in,
- the people we see every day,
- the clothes we wear, and
- the health we have.

Here is a short story that I love that really expresses our need for being grateful every day:

A blind boy sat on the steps of a building with a hat by his feet. He held up a sign which read, "I am blind, please help." There were only a few coins thrown in the hat—spare change from people as they hurried past.

A man was walking by. He took a few coins from his pocket and dropped them into the hat. He then took the sign, turned it around, and wrote some words. Then he put the sign back in the boy's hand so that everyone that passed by would see the new words.

Soon the hat began to fill up. A lot more people were giving money to the blind boy. That afternoon, the man who had changed the sign returned to see how things were. The boy recognized his cologne and asked, "Were you the one who changed my sign this morning? What did you write?"

"I only wrote the truth," the man responded. "I said what you said, but differently. I wrote, 'Today is a beautiful day, but I cannot see it.'"

Both signs spoke the truth, but the first sign simply said the boy was blind, while the second sign conveyed to everyone walking by how grateful they should be to see.

When things begin to feel stressful and out of control, it always seems challenging to maintain an attitude of gratitude. What we see at that moment of turmoil is just that—turmoil. That kind of view, however, is very harmful to how upbeat we feel throughout the day.

There is nothing wrong with being appreciative or blissful about those things we get that comes to use seldom: a new car, a job offer at multibillion-dollar companies, admission to an Ivy League college, but we shouldn't take granted the everyday things we have: our health, family, clothes, the food we eat, and the water we drink. We often take these precious commodities for granted. Meanwhile, the things we take for granted are usually the things we can't do without, such as water, food, and family. Caught up in the bliss, comfort, and familiarity of it all, we can simply forget to be thankful.

Before you complain about not having enough, ask yourself these questions, Have I been grateful for my health? Have I been thankful for the car(s) I have? Have I been grateful for the meal I had? Have I been grateful for the life of my children? Have I been thankful for my body? Have I been grateful for the supportive friends and family I have?

Think about that.

Expressing gratitude doesn't have to be you receiving things from others, but it can also come from you showing acts of kindness to others—stranger or not.

There are various acts of kindness that you can do, which won't cost much.

- Bring toys to the homeless shelter,
- hold the elevator door for someone,
- give strangers compliments,
- make a music playlist for someone,
- help someone put groceries in their car,
- bake cookies for the office,
- read a book to an older adult,
- give your favourite book to a friend,
- buy the person behind you coffee,
- send love notes to your spouse,
- pick up litter at the park,
- shake hand with kids and adults,
- donate to a charity,
- wash someone's dishes, or do someone a favour.

These are acts of kindness that cost little to nothing; that would not just bring happiness to the person you are doing it to but also make you happy. There was a day I was heading home from work when I saw a grown woman. She was hauling a nylon bag that I noticed looked like it was about to tear. At first, I didn't think it would be an issue, but a few minutes later, the bag got wholly torn. All the fruits and veggies she had put into it fell to the ground and got scattered. When I witnessed this event, I took it upon myself to help the senior. After picking all the scattered fruits and veggies for her, she exuded gratitude. She thanked and hugged me and also gave me fruit as well. The smiles on her face made me happy. It felt good.

Studies have shown, when people express help to others, the recipients are also likely to do the same to others. Generosity is contagious. Gratitude can be thought of as a medicine that strengthens you mentally, physically, and socially. People who are more thankful experience more energy, handle stress better, eat healthier diets, have deeper friendships, have increased self-worth, enjoy work and perform better on the job, sleep better, handle challenges better, and are more optimistic. That's a lot of good stuff.

Here are some of the activities you could do to make gratitude a part of your every day and relish some of its benefits:

1. *Tell someone you appreciate them.* Smile more often; avoid negative media and contents; volunteer for organizations that help others; focus on your strength, commit a day in a week when you won't complain about anything.

2. *Tell your family how much you love and appreciate them.* When you are at home, thank your spouse for the effort and support they've added in keeping the family afloat. Say thank you to your children for being a good listener and for helping mow the lawn. You could send your wife flowers or something as simple as respect. Take your children to the park, watch the latest blockbuster movie, or you could get them something they love. This is to show that you acknowledge them and their importance in your life.

3. *Smile more often.* Smiling to people doesn't just give you a feeling of happiness, but it does the same for the other person. When you smile at people, they make themselves more open and vulnerable because they couldn't pick up any signs of a threat from you. This practice increases the length and intimacy of conversations and fosters a stronger bond between both parties. From this time forth, smile to everyone you associate with—the cabman, the shopkeeper, the librarian, friends, and even those you dislike; it might just change them.

4. *Avoid harmful media content.* Stop yourself from consuming negative and violent contents from the news networks. The information you consume would determine the way you interpret the world. Your mind is like a factory. The ingredients you put into it will be used to make the final product—your life. Always sought after positive content that is inspirational, motivating, and uplifting. Remember: It is what you feed that will grow. So, feed your mind with positive information.

5. *Focus on your strength.* Realizing that you can't have everything you want and that you aren't perfect, can be the best discovery to becoming happy. Rather than focusing on your failure or weakness, invest your energy into your success and strength. Knowing what you are good at and being confident at it builds self-esteem. Should you focus on the negatives of life, you will be doing yourself a disservice, as it would make you feel weak, lose self-worth, and lose the respect others have for you. Note this: Focus on the possibilities of success, not on the potential for failure.

6. *Commit a day in a week when you won't complain about anything.* Schedule, at least, a day each week to allow yourself to experience poise, serenity, and the positiveness of life. You can use this period to meditate as well. It helps you become more self-aware, relaxed and makes you experience more positivity out of life. Use this period to focus on all the good that has happened to you in the past few days, weeks, and months, and then build on it.

7. *Volunteer your time to help others.* Things as paltry as holding the elevator door, running errands for someone, mowing your neighbour's lawn, and sending a care package to a soldier can go a great length in allowing others to develop trust and increase their respect for you.

Let's all live the words of John F. Kennedy: "As we express our gratitude, we must never forget that the highest appreciation is not to utter words, but to live by them."

Life has a positive meaning

Life is beautiful, and its host (humans, and possibly aliens) are created for a purpose. We tend not to attach meaning to life and think that the negative events that happen in our lives are based on bad luck. Well, that might not be true.

Everything in life has its cause and meaning. We feel the way we think because of the emotions we created and how we interpret them. These chronic emotional feelings (feelings of emptiness and meaninglessness) can cause depression, loneliness, addiction and aggression. And one of the best methods to alleviate such emotional feelings is to attach a positive meaning to them.

When I was younger, like most kids, I always wanted new shoes and clothes. My parents, however, didn't have much but always made sure to feed the home. Not having enough resources to get what you want is an unpleasant experience for any kid, primarily when they associate themselves with friends who has a lot of things.

I always complained. My parents didn't have enough money to enrol me in the right school. I hardly went out with my friends because I had no proper clothes. These challenges were tough on me, but little did I know that it would cause a monumental change.

As days, months, and years grew, these trails and pain made me stronger. Because of my hunger to have money to feed my family and become successful, I began the journey of self-development. I read books on wealth and success, and I also adopted patience. I developed self-awareness and empathy. And it is what led me to write this book you are now reading. Understanding the meaning of your pain and suffering is an essential step to becoming happier.

"To live is to suffer, to survive is to find meaning in the suffering. If there is a purpose in life at all, there must be a purpose in suffering and dying." – Excerpt of *Man's Search for Meaning*.

Here is a story of a man in *Man's Search for Meaning* by Viktor Frankl, who found meaning in his suffering:

```
Once, an elderly general practitioner consulted me because of his
severe depression. He could not overcome the loss of his wife,
who had died two years before and whom he had loved above all
else. Now, how could I help him? What should I tell him? Well, I
refrained from telling him anything but instead confronted him
with the question, "What would have happened, Doctor, if you had
died first, and your wife would have had to survive you?" "Oh,"
he said, "for her, this would have been terrible; how she would
have suffered!" I replied, "You see Doctor, such a suffering has
```

```
been spared her, and you who have spared her this suffering to be
sure at the price that you now have to survive and mourn her." He
said no word but shook my hand, and calmly left my office.
```

In some way, suffering ceases to be suffering the moment it finds a meaning, such as the meaning of a sacrifice. Realizing that no one is immune to pain and the only way to curb it is to attach a positive connotation to it so you can be happy. Everyone feels the pain of some sort; even the millionaires and billionaires you see and watch on TV all feel pain. Their pains might not come from lack of money or cars, but it might be from their marriage, children, friends, family, or their sinking business sales. You might not have money now, but you probably have good children who care and love you; family and friends that would always stand by your side and support you; or a loving relationship with your spouse that brings joy to you every day.

These words might sound like cliché—No pain, No gain—but it is true. The soreness you face in your marriage or business can motivate and strengthen you to find a way to save your marriage or make you associate with people who have experience in building a successful business, respectively.

The pain I felt, is what pushed me to find meaningful ways to spend my time and energy on activities that are productive and important to helping me become fiscally stable and creative. Here are two thoughts about pain and suffering you should know about:

First, pain is an opportunity for growth. If you can, I want you to thoughtfully pick a person on this planet Earth who is successful that hasn't or won't feel pain in their entire life. Anybody? I doubt you will find one. This world is built on pain. You can't dodge it. You can't hide from it, but you can embrace it, and only those who embrace pain are sure to be transformed. The reason people crave a good relationship is, perhaps, because of the pain we've felt when we were in a bad relationship. The pain makes us desire better for ourselves.

If you've never been to a gym, then I recommend you do so. When you go to a gym and try to work out, you will feel pain, without a doubt. Your hands will become sore, your tummy will cramp, salty water will drip out of your body, and your heartbeat will grow faster as blood rushes through your body, providing oxygen to every part of your muscle. Your body will scream, PAIN! But the result, as you might know, over weeks and months of effort, would become visible in the form of a body transformation—more muscular abs, bigger muscles, broad chest, and greater fitness.

We all know about this, but most of us don't want to put in the sacrifice it takes. We don't want to feel pain. Only those who choose to embrace and work with pain; are the people who make real success and happiness. For those who embrace pain, the fun part is: the result of pain is usually apparent. If you walk on the street and notice a lady who is fit with abs and excellent flexibility, it would tell you that the lady does workout. A kid who answers most exam questions would mean that he or she has spent more time reading than his or her peers.

Here is a list of people who felt pain and suffering before they became successful: Steve Harvey, Tony Robbins, Oprah Winfrey, Elon Musk, JK Rowlings, Stephen King, Bill Gates, Mark Wahlberg, Mariah Carey. Here is a list of companies that started very little, but are now a multibillion-dollar company: Coca-Cola, Hewlett-Packard (HP), Starbucks, Apple, Microsoft, Netflix, Mattel, Spanx, McDonald's.

Do you see the point here? In the beginning, what life throws at you is usually tough, but if you hang on there's always a positive meaning and result behind those hurdles.

Second, pain is temporary. I don't know what situation you are in or the trials you are facing now, but here is what I know; it will pass. Nothing is constant. In fact, change is the only constant thing in life. Emotion changes, the weather changes, the government changes, law changes, and people change. What you feel right now would not last forever; it's only there for a moment. Here is a story of Joseph:

When Joseph lost his mother at the age of twenty-seven, he cried, he wallowed in misery. He couldn't eat or drink. He felt all alone during this period.

"How can I survive without my mother," he said wallowing.

A day after his mother's death, I went to visit him at home. I met him on the couch in tears and worries. I asked him, "Why are you crying? Your cries won't help the situation."

"Why won't I ?" he answered in a deep, sorrowful voice. "I just lost my mother. I have no one with me. How am I going to survive without my mother?"

I understood his pain, all children rely on their parents (mothers especially), but I told him, "You aren't alone; you still have your father and your elder brothers around you. They also grief, but they understand that they have to move on with their lives. Thinking about your mom all day would only cause harm to your health. So cheer up."

Two weeks later, he came home with smiles and joy when he relayed the news that he had been appointed to work in an investment bank that he had previously done an interview for. The next day, he came to my apartment to inform me about the good news. I saw his face beaming with happiness and joy.

I was happy for him.

But I told him, "When you were in tears about your mom's death, didn't I tell you to cheer up that all would be well?" "Yes, you did," he responded. "I was influenced by my emotions. I didn't notice that I was surrounded by a great family who would always love and support me just as my mother did love me."

Though Joseph lost his mother, his life wasn't any worse as he thought. When you are in a state of pain, always remember: it is temporary. The pain will pass and be patient. Always attach positive meaning to your predicaments that can help build confidence in yourself. For example:

1. Rather than seeing yourself as a failure when you failed a test, instead, think of it as an opportunity for you to study harder and be better prepared for the next one.
2. Rather than feeling bad for your best friend deserting you, instead, think of it as a way to become more dependent on yourself.
3. Rather than complaining about why you got fired at work or how your boss is nuts, instead, think of it as an opportunity to think creatively so

you can have your own business.

Many of our stress, aggression, and depression would be reduced or gone if only we can think and see the positive in our situations. As Chuck Swindoll said, "Life is 10 percent what happens to you and 90 percent how you react to it." To put it better: Life is more about the meaning you give to it. Remember: when you feel depressed, angry, or stressed, take a minute to think, and ask yourself what meaning you attach to the pains you feel.

Focus On Here and Now

There are two groups of chemicals in your brain that control your experience of satisfaction: the down and up chemicals, as referred to in the book, *The Molecule of More* by Daniel Lieberman. The up chemicals or neurotransmitters (as they're often called) allows you to pursue things beyond your immediate grasp, but it also motivates you. It drives you to appreciate and seek out those things that are far away, including things you can't see, such as love and power. Whether it's reaching for the moon, winning a Nobel Prize, becoming a president, inventing a new technology, or finding the cure to a disease, this chemical makes you chase it because of the distant reward you might get. It makes you want more; however, it never gives you real satisfaction.

The down chemical that Lieberman refers to as "Here & Now" allows you to appreciate what's in your current domain—the things you have now. This chemical makes you focus on your surroundings and enables you to relish what you have and see. But it also triggers the fight-or-flight response to flee from dangers now. As Daniel Z. Lieberman wrote: "The up chemical makes you desire what you don't yet have, and drives you to seek new things. It rewards you when you obey it and makes you suffer when you don't. It is the source of creativity and, further along the spectrum, madness; it is the key to addiction and the path to recovery."

These two chemicals are the reasons for our wants and desires. The down chemical allows you to experience what is close, while the up chemical gives you the craving to pursue what is far away. It would be much easier for you to achieve happiness and satisfaction right now if you could appreciate and focus on what you have today, rather than on what you don't have or who you could be tomorrow.

In our current world, where we are told what to do, what not to do, what to have, and what not to have, it can become distracting to be our true self. We tend to do things we don't feel comfortable about because everyone else is doing the same. We lose ourselves trying to become someone else in the process. You are convinced by the constant bombardment of advertisements on TV, radio, billboard, magazine, telling you that you are not enough or can't be enough until you buy their product or service. It would be a journey leading to a path of dissatisfaction and unhappiness. These are two things you should focus on that would help you bring back happiness into your life.

Remember Those Close To You: Friends and Family

It is surprising how we tend not to be appreciative of our family and friends—your children who always bring joy to your heart, your spouse that gives you massages when you come home tired and stressed; friends that help in completing some of your work, or even your maids who help in taking care of the home—Yes, even though you pay them. Your family should be one of the first sources of joy. Even in the modern world, with the advancement of technologies, new forms of communication, and changing cultural norms, having a family is just as important as it ever was. No matter how much life changes in the future, it will probably continue to be needed in one way or another.

In general terms, a family consists of two parents and their children living together as a unit. Aunts, uncles, cousins, and grandparents might live together within the same household or not, albeit, that practice isn't as common in recent times. The extended family system is still widely practised in some parts of Asia: China, India, Malaysia, but these have become less popular in western culture. Now, a family can consist of two or more parents of any gender, married or not. The children may have been born to one of the parents, both parents, or adopted.

Families are of importance to society and people's lives. They teach us a lot about life and relationships. Families can be a source of support to help us weather life's changes and challenges. Below are some of the benefits of having a family.

1. *The family meets physical and emotional needs.* Families help provide basic needs such as water, food, and shelter to the other family members. This creates a special bond amongst members to support each other during times of difficulty. Moreover, a family cares for our emotional needs as well. Many years ago, Abram Maslow formed a psychological concept called *Maslow's Hierarchy of Needs,* to help us understand which needs are essential to us. Maslow's Hierarchy of Needs has a pyramid structure, with the broad base of the pyramid representing our basic needs such as water, air, sleep, and shelter. These are things that are most important to our survival. The next three levels are the needs our family can provide us with to reach the peak of Maslow's pyramid—self-actualization.

2. *Safety needs.* Once our physiological needs are satisfied, the need for our security and safety becomes essential. Things such as personal security, employment, resources, health, and property can be provided to us with our family and society's help. A family should provide financial protection for everyone living in the household. Both parents should assist themselves in paying the bills and providing the children with proper education. Society can help provide the necessary safety needs for the growth of people through job employment, appropriate medical care by the doctors, adequate training by the teachers, and security by police.

3. *Love and belongings.* Once our physiological and safety needs have been met, the third level of human need involves a sense of belonging. Families are essential in helping children meet these needs. Through daily socialization and interaction, parents can help their children feel valued, loved, and wanted. Friends also could help in this development by actively expressing interest for each other and giving or receiving affection from one another. Healthy families always have each other's

back and feelings of concern for a member when they notice signs of distress or anxiety.

4. *Health benefits.* According to a research study published by Harvard Health Publishing, people who have children are more likely to live longer than those who are childless. And this could be because people with children may have healthier habits—less smoking, less alcohol, more physical activity than those who are childless. People with children tend to have more social interactions with other parents than those without a child. Children in a healthy family tend to enjoy tasty meals, spend more time outdoors, receive better education, and the right medical care when needed.

5. *Community benefits.* Children from a proper home are taught to contribute more to society than they take from it. They are trained to be generous to other people. They volunteer their time and resources—money, prayers, and food to help support and grow the community, helping the current and future generations to come. Because of the diversity of a city, children could tend to learn different skills or discover what they like or want to do as a career based on the people they associate themselves with. Residents of a positive community can help support each other's needs (i.e., protecting each other's houses, taking care of children when their parents are not around) and desires.

6. *Family helps develop self-esteem.* A healthy family helps their children develop self-confidence, strength, freedom, respect, and recognition by giving children essential responsibilities and involving them in relevant family decisions. By giving children the liberty to speak their minds and concern, you help foster self-esteem, which is vital in the development of a child. Maintaining self-confidence is essential to become confident at the workplace, to build a healthier relationship, to experience happiness and gratitude, and be open to learning and feedback, which can help you acquire and master new skills.

The role of family should be: to love, respect each other, encourage, support, and build each other. A family that cannot do this is not just damaging the children's morale, but it also fosters a corrupt society that evolves into creating a corrupt country.

Remember the Good Experience Not the Bad

One of the problems we have, as humans, is that people tend to focus more on their failures than their successes. It's said that we have around 60,000 thoughts per day, and eighty percent of those thoughts are negative—dead weights. Whenever we experience a negative situation or a problem, we feel sad and cry about it for days, weeks, and months. But when something good happens to us, we celebrate and enjoy it for about a day or two.

What does this mean?

We often remember the bad experience more than a pleasant experience. This kind of thought is harmful to you emotionally and psychologically. The pains, suffering, and harrowing experience you remember would consume you and leave you needing help to become psychologically stable. You will most likely remember the day you got your graduation or the day of your honeymoon far less than the day you had an accident that nearly left you crippled.

The mind tends to hold longer onto experiences that made you fear, caused you pain, or made you fight or flee, than the positive experiences that brought you happiness, raised your spirit, or made you cry tears of joy. Positive thoughts create positive people, not necessarily a positive experience. You don't need to have a good experience before you can think positively. Your thought is a choice. Whatever your beliefs are—negative or positive—it's your choice to make.

So, it is possible to have a bad experience but still have a good day. Do you remember the part where we talked about attaching a positive meaning to your painful experience? That is what you need to do. A student who just failed a class test, rather than complaining about how unfair the teacher was, should spend his "thought energy" thinking of ways to spend more time reading, to become better prepared. For a lady who just got fired at her workplace, instead of cussing and complaining about how lame her boss is, she should spend her "thought energy" focusing on the reasons she was fired in the first place and what she can do to avoid that from happening again. Rather than focusing on what your spouse could not do well, focus your "thought energy" on what you are not good at and become good at it so that your spouse can have the urge also to change. You'll never feel good about yourself unless you focus and appreciate the good memories you have.

Whenever you feel moody or downcast, try to focus on the positive experience. If you feed the beast, it will consume you. Here are a few things you could always do to bring yourself back to a state of bliss.

1. *Identify your areas of negativity.* Identify the cause of the negative feeling and tackle the depressing thoughts to bring you to resolve. For the student who feels distressed for failing the test, he should not spend time wallowing; instead, he should spend time to understand the questions he failed. For the lady who felt sad from being sacked from work, she should inquire about her boss or work colleague what she had done wrong and what she could do to improve. The husband, who always complains about the wife not doing enough, should clearly, without anger, explain his realistic expectations from her, and he should also ask her what she expects from him, and they should both work on it.

2. *Spend time with positive people.* It's often said that we are an average of the five people we associate with. Spending a lot of your time with positive people would allow for more positive experiences and make you a positive person. Positive friends could help you see the fun part of the world rather than that often portrayed by the media.

3. *Start your day on a positive note.* Before going to work each day, always say five positive words to yourself. "I am happy." "Today is going to be awesome." "I am filled with a positive vibe." "I have all it takes." "I am capable of ..." Make sure to exercise regularly for at least ten minutes. And always choose to eat healthy diets. Say thank you to the provider of the food and to the one who cooked it—and if that's you, pat yourself at the back.

4. *Keep a gratitude journal.* Before going to bed for the day, make sure to

write down at least ten positive things that you experienced. Having a gratitude journal is a significant thing to do to keep you positive always. It helps you remember positive memories. And when you can't find anything positive about a day, your gratitude journal can act as a bank that stores "gratitude currency" that you can take to refill your positivity bar.

5. *Meditate.* Meditation has been proven to help people become happier by focusing their thoughts on positive experiences. All you need to practice meditation is a soft floor and a relatively quiet place. Meditation can help you become more focused on your surroundings and less agitated when faced with a negative experience.

In modern society, where there is rampant dissatisfaction in jobs, homes, schools, and politics, it has become a significant priority to make people understand that there's a lot to be thankful for to help pour happiness into their lives. Commit these words of Lao Tzu, "If you are depressed, you are living in the past. If you are anxious, you are living in the future. If you are at peace, you are living in the present."

4

Principle #4: Grow Your Mind and Body

Strive not to be a success, but rather to be of value. — Albert Einstein.

Have you ever asked yourself these questions: Am I working on my short- and long-term goals? Are these foods healthy for me? What steps can I take to be in good shape and mindset? These are personal development questions we need to ask ourselves daily. Without these questions, how can you know if you are improving on a particular section of your life? Personal development is a vital process to self-improvement in our dynamic, fast-paced world. As we move through life, we are guaranteed to face diverse circumstances, changing environments, and new roles that require our utmost strength to adapt. Personal development allows for the improvement of awareness and identity, develops talents and skills, and increases the quality of life and contributes to the realization of dreams and aspirations.

Personal development enhances your self-confidence to a new level. It also presents you with new opportunities when you spend time and energy developing yourself in a particular skill you could get paid for in a needed market. The ultimate benefit of self-improvement is for you to become a better version of yourself. Realizing who you are and what your capabilities are, is essential in the process of helping you understand your true self. Growth is necessary (if not the most important) in every aspect of your life—workplace, relationship, family, and education. Self-improvement helps you set priorities and put plans in place to achieve a remarkable level of success.

There are various ways self-improvement can help positively affect your life:

First, it helps develop self-esteem. Finding strategies to improve yourself by growing and learning every day can help boost your confidence. Self-improvement enables you to identify what you're weak at and lets you upgrade to become better. The more you keep developing yourself in the areas of your life you are weak at, the more growth you will promote.

Second, it increases your self-awareness. Knowing what you are good and weak at is an essential quality of self-improvement. It helps you understand yourself better by questioning yourself and face reality for what it is, however harsh it might be. Self-awareness is an ongoing journey that never stops as life progresses. You will experience different adversities and challenges, thoughts and feelings, making self-improvement even more important to never lose touch with yourself.

Why Reading Is Important

That's the thing about books. They let you travel without moving your feet. — Jhumpa Lahiri.

You've read books at some point in your life, and you are reading one right now. Reading a book is arguably the most crucial skill for developing oneself. Reading has a lot of good things to offer. It has been shown to prevent Alzheimer's, improve concentration, help with depression, and enhance self-confidence. According to Cristle Russell, a behavioural researcher, reading can reduce the presence of stress and turmoil. Each book that you read helps you to understand the world better and learn something new. Whether you are out of college, or still in a relationship, or working in a nine-to-five job, everyone needs information to consume. Reading is one of the best forms of self-education for both children and adults, too.

People who choose not to read tend to be ignorant of themselves, their friends, and the world. A world without readers would mean a world with an increase in stress level, less creativity and research, low self-esteem, and compassion. Reading also creates millionaires and billionaires that provide the poor with donations and reduces violence as poverty lowers.

How Books Evolved

Before the creation of books, humans communicated through the use of cave drawings and words—that is, storytelling. Storytelling was one of the ways our ancestors entertained and taught lessons about the danger of the woods to the tribe. It was how fairy tales began and how language and spoken words found their power. Cave drawings were one of the ways the archaic civilization communicated and recorded their lives.

But, before we dive in deeper, what, really, is a book?

In a few words, a book is a written or printed literary work. In archaic days, different materials were used for books, such as bamboo and beech bark. As books evolved and became cheaper, they became a widespread means of conveying and storing information.

The ancient Egyptians were the first to use scrolls. A scroll was a rolled manuscript made by weaving together stems of the papyrus plant, then flattening the twisted stems by pounding them flat. The Greeks and Romans adopted this method until the 8th century AD. The Romans later created "the codex," which was bound and opened up like a book with pages. This became widely used as it was less likely to tear. The pages were made from parchments, such as calfskin or deerskin. The Romans added a table of contents and indexes. Since the codex was portable and easy to travel with, the early Christians adopted it to travel with it in distant lands. The Greeks and Romans invented the tablets, which were blocks of wood that layered with wax so you could scratch a message into them, then erase and re-use them again and again.

Printed Books

According to historical sources, the Han dynasty Chinese court official, Cal Lun, invented the first paper made with plant fibers. In AD 868, the Chinese nation made the first and indeed printed book called the Diamond Sutra. But it was not until the Gutenberg printing press that writing could be published more quickly. Before Johannes Gutenberg built the world's first-ever printing press or movable type, only the wealthy could afford the use of books. The Gutenberg Bible was the first book (and the oldest surviving printed book) that Gutenberg printed that was mass-produced. With the invention of the printing press, people began to buy and read more books as literature began to flourish. Reference books like dictionaries also became popular. Pamphlets were also printed. Pamphlets later led to magazines and newspapers—the two primary means of conveying information today.

In the 19th century, aspiring publishers started printing hardback books aimed at wealthier people with the idea that hardbacks were thought to be great works of fine literature, and paperbacks were considered silly. Two American brothers named Boni created a publishing company that sent books by mail order. Eventually, it became Random House. The Boni brothers were closely followed in 1935 by Penguin. This successful British publisher printed beautiful branded books that appealed to everyone. This created the dawn of the publishing formats such as audiobooks and the eBook or kindle.

Effects of Reading Books

Reading books, at least one complete book a month or twelve books a year, has been proven to aid in developing the brain—mentally and emotionally, and how we socialize with our environment. Below are the ways reading improves our mental and physical health.

1. *It improves your vocabulary.* Reading exposes you to more words, which allows for understanding terms and concepts in different ways. Reading an hour a day exposes you to about four million words per year. Research

has shown that it is crucial to begin reading from a young age. Children who read books more often, starting from a young age, gradually develop large vocabularies. Having a large number of vocabularies can influence specific areas of your life, from being able to articulate yourself socially, to getting more significant job opportunities, and improving your standardized test scores. A 2019 survey, conducted by Cengage, showed that a study of more than 650 employers revealed that "soft" skills are most in-demand by at least sixty-five percent of the employer; above quantitative skills (forty-seven percent) and computer and technical skills (fifty percent).

2. *It helps reduce depression.* In a study, conducted by the University of Liverpool, four to eight voluntary adult participants partook in a two-weekly reading group, that resulted in significant improvement in the mental health of depressed patients during the twelve-month period in which they had attended the reading group. Reading fiction books can lessen the feeling of being isolated, which is one of the causes of depression by escaping your world into the domain of the author's imagination. And in nonfiction, self-help books, you can learn different ways to manage or prevent mental illness.

3. *It enables you to connect with and understand people.* Reading an autobiography about someone can help you understand the life of the person and lessons from their life experience that you could implement into your life. Learning about other people's cultures and countries without being there physically can help you understand and appreciate their lifestyle. Reading books on how to connect and socialize with others can teach you the strategies and ways to associate with others in a friendly manner.

4. *It reduces stress.* A 2009 study report on the immediate effect of yoga, humour, and reading, on acute stress in students, showed that a thirty-minute session of yoga, fun, and reading had a similar impact in decreasing severe stress in health science students. It is a critical study as it could allow educators and psychologists to begin to consider different stress strategies for managing the stress of people.

5. *Increases survival rate.* A 2007 study, published by NCBI, reported a group

that consisted of 3,635 participants in the nationally representative Health and Retirement Study (HRS) showed that compared to non-book readers, book readers had a four months survival advantage; and also experienced a twenty percent reduced risk of mortality over the twelve years of follow up compared to non-book readers.

6. *It improves your sleep.* A few minutes of reading at night can help you sleep better. A study from the University of Sussex found that reading helps to alleviate insomnia. If you have trouble sleeping at night, make sure to use a print book rather than reading from your device. The light from the screen has been proven to suppress melatonin—a hormone that regulates the sleep-wake cycle.

Now that you know the psychological and physical advantageous effect that reading provides, it is time you understand some of the ways to cultivate the habit of reading often. As Somerset Maugham said: To acquire the habit of reading is to construct for yourself a refuge from almost all the miseries of life.

1. *Find a quiet place to read.* Having a quiet place to read at home, work, or school during breaks, away from a noisy family member or roommates, is vital to creating a special glue with the books you read. Wherever you choose to read, make sure it's free from objects that could cause distraction—computer, TV, phones, and laptops.

2. *Schedule times for reading.* When you consciously set a time for reading, it gives you a sense of direction and focus. Rather than saying, "I am going to read today," instead, say to yourself, "Today, I am going to be reading [the name of the book] from 4 pm to 5 pm, at this study room." It is more specific, which raises the chances of you reading. And it doesn't have to be an hour read. Depending on how the day is, you can decide to read for ten minutes or more.

3. *Always carry a book.* There is a thing I learned from Bill Gates: he still takes at least a book wherever he goes. Like the way you move your phone or favourite gadget wherever you go, you should do the same

with books. When you are in traffic, in order not to waste precious time, make sure to spend your traffic time listening to audiobooks or reading printed books. Whether it is to a meeting, to a school, or an event, make sure to take at least one form of a book—audiobooks, eBook, or printed book—with you so that you make good use of the breaks or delays you might have.

4. *Make a list of books to read each month.* Keep a list of all the books you want to read. Whenever you hear about a good book either on TV, or online, or in person, make sure to write it down in a pocket notebook, a journal, on your homepage, or whatever means you prefer. If you are more serious about it, you can give yourself a specific number and names of books you must finish within a month and then cross out those you read from your list.

What Seminars Can Offer

It is not just important to learn from textbooks alone. Attending seminars can help you achieve success in your academic environment by utilizing your skill in real-world practice. A seminar or workshop is a conference that involves a group of people led by an expert that focuses on specific themes or disciplines such as marketing, business, networking, or a university field. Seminars typically take place over a few days. They can involve corporate discussion, multiple speakers, and opportunities to share perspectives and issues related to the topic.

For a student who needs more than just knowledge from a textbook, but wants a more collaborative and hands-on type of expertise with present participants, led by a real expert in their discipline, seminars can be the best option. Seminars provide in-depth knowledge about a specific topic as they can ask questions, and take notes. The student doesn't just receive detailed information from experts. They also have the opportunity to meet other people who share your interest, allowing for an exchange of knowledge between attendees. The relationship you build with the attendees can continue into your personal and professional life even after the seminar has ended.

Attending seminars also helps improve communication skills and allows you to present your argument and ideas to attendees and experts.

Webinars have become one of the most popular uses of interacting with people and learning from experts from your home's comfort. A webinar is the online transmission of seminars, presentations, or similar content through the internet. It is the combination of the word "web" and "seminar." As of the time of this writing, we face a global pandemic that has increased the global use of online video transmission in the education and business sectors. The advancement and extensive use of this technology has made it easy to share contents, such as videos and images online to people who have now accepted and adopted the use of live streaming content for conferences, live webcasts, seminars, business, and schools.

Before starting a webinar, a start and end time is usually given in advance, as it can be taking place in real-time or recorded so that it can be downloaded later. In the webinar, participants and speakers don't have to be in the same room to interact and share information. Depending on the organizer, participants could be given the right to speak, chat, share a file, and conduct surveys directly.

Here are some of the benefits of webinars:

- Attendees are allowed to participate anonymously.
- Easy to exchange information before, during, and after the event.
- It enables participants to share or download additional digital materials during the webinar.
- Less costly as there's no need to travel or book a hotel.
- Since participants are not in a room confined to the number of seats, they could be as much as 10,000 participants.

Why You Need Healthy Eating and Regular Exercise

You've probably heard from friends, families, magazines, or TV about the importance of having a healthy diet. Eating healthy foods and drinks is, without a doubt, good for the body and mental development. A healthy diet doesn't just require the consumption of a specific type of nutrients, but it involves the use of the various kinds of nutrients—vitamins, protein, fat, carbohydrate, etc.—at their moderate levels. A person that practices a daily healthy diet would develop a much strengthened immune system, better mental growth, a healthy heart, strong bones, healthy muscles.

According to a report by the World Health Organization (WHO), healthy nutrition increases the lifespan of a person and reduces the risk of disability from major nutrition-related chronic diseases. Continuous practice of poor diet can lead to or contribute to high blood pressure, dental infections, osteoporosis, heart disease, stroke, several forms of cancer, and obesity.

According to the Center for Disease Control and Prevention (CDC) report from 1999-2000 through 2017-2018, the number of obese people increased from 30.5 percent to 42.4 percent, and an increase in severe obesity from 4.7 percent to 9.2 percent. The rise of obesity has become a significant epidemic challenge facing doctors today (both literally and figuratively). The estimated annual medical cost of obesity in the United States was $147 billion in 2008. The increase in the consumption of extreme fatty food or Trans fatty acid (TFAs), junk foods, sugar (fructose and glucose), and less physical activity has contributed to the rise of obesity.

Although obesity in itself is not a disease as it arises from having too much energy. It has been a significant contributor to the surge of other forms of illness such as cardiovascular disease, stroke, type 2 diabetes, cancer, nonalcoholic fatty liver disease. An individual with a body mass index (BMI) greater than $30Kg/m^2$ is said to be obese.

According to the National Institutes of Health, obesity and overweight are the second leading cause of preventable deaths per year in the United States. Since the 1970s, the number of obese people has doubled, with about two-thirds of adults in the U.S. are obese, and one-third of the children are overweight. But why the increase of obesity and its related disease, when it can be prevented? First, we have to know how the body stores and uses energy for our daily use.

How the Body Stores and Use Energy

When we walk, run, sleep, swim, or lift weights, we spend energy that is being produced by the food we consume. All parts of our body (muscle, brain, heart) need continuous power to work or function properly. The need for energy is for the growth and reproduction of the cells. As you ingest food, numerous metabolic reactions begin to occur inside the cells that would later produce water, carbon dioxide, and a chemical energy called Adenosine triphosphate (ATP). These metabolic reactions are essential to life as your cells would die if they stop. ATP molecules are often referred to as the "molecular unit currency," as they provide the energy necessary to drive many processes in a living cell such as muscle contraction, breathing, nerve impulse propagation, and chemical synthesis.

ATP helps to store and transport chemical energy with cells when needed. In turn, your body synthesizes and recharges ATP molecules by burning fuel, mostly fats, carbohydrates, and sometimes proteins. So, ATP can be looked at as a battery that helps store energy gotten from the foods you eat and sends those energies to wherever it is needed in your body—just as the way you charge your phone when you notice the battery energy is depleted from the use of it. Our daily food choices resupply the potential energy or fuel that the body requires to function normally. The body can store some of the fuels in various forms—triglycerides, and glycogen—that offers the muscles a constant supply of energy.

When there is an excess source of fuel, the body converts them and stores them into muscle, liver, and fat cells. Too many of these nutrients do harm the body. For example, a person who consumes too many carbohydrates and fats develop storage cells in the body that help store excess energy. Because people do less exercising and less energy-intensive work due to the increase of technology and automation, it allows for the accumulation of unused energy in us that could have been spent while working. This built-up energy stays in our body, and later becomes a problem that can lead to various illnesses.

A very high protein diet overworks the liver and kidney cells, as they need to brake the excess nutrients and excrete them. These organs become damaged, causing illness or early death. The body burns carbohydrate quicker and much easier than fats, but carbs store energy less densely. A gram of carbs contains four calories, a gram of protein contains four calories, and a gram of fat contains nine calories. The surprising thing about this is: the things that cause more harm to our health (i.e., sugar and saturated fats) are becoming cheaper than the foods that are healthy to consume, as technology helps to increase productivity and reduce manufacturing cost. Saturated fats or low-density lipoprotein fats (LDL) are bad cholesterols that instigate the liver to produce unhealthier LDLs. Saturated fats are used in many packaged foods, which increase the risk of weight gain, heart disease, stroke, and block blood vessels.

It is estimated that the average person in the United States consumes around 19.5 teaspoons or eighty-two grams of sugar per day. That is over double the amount recommended by the American Heart Association (AHA), which is nine teaspoons per day for men and six teaspoons for women. Consuming too much sugar increases your risk of having type 2 diabetes, heart disease, infections, and kidney disease. Maintaining a healthy weight and increasing physical activity plays a vital role in the prevention and treatment of diabetes.

Cardiovascular disease, a worldwide health problem, is caused due to physical inactivity and poor nutrition. Maintaining a proper diet of fruits, vegetables, eating less saturated fat, and less intake salt helps reduce blood pressure, a significant cause of cardiovascular disease. Several forms of cancers are contributed significantly by dietary factors. A healthy diet of reducing your alcohol intake and tobacco (the number one leading cause of cancer) will limit the risk of cancer of the mouth, liver, breast, kidney, and oesophagus. A healthy diet of fruit, vegetable, and exercise promotes a healthy sex life, strengthen the immune systems, and lower your risk of breast, uterine, and colorectal cancer.

Dental diseases are caused by excess consumption of carbohydrates (sugar and starch) such as milk, soda, and fruits and dietary acids in beverages and other acidic foods. In your mouth, lots of bacteria feast on the munched pieces of diet for their growth and produce acid, which dissolves the enamel, creating holes in the teeth called cavities. You can limit the risk of dental disease by flossing your teeth daily with fluoride-containing toothpaste and visiting the dentist at least once a year.

Eating and drinking more than your body needs creates an opportunity for your body to gain weight because the energy you don't use is stored as fat in the body. If you eat and drink too little, you'll lose weight. Knowing the kinds of food you should eat, and how much you should eat, what to drink, and how much to drink is essential to having a healthy lifestyle. Here are some practical things you can do to begin a healthy eating lifestyle.

1. *Eat lots of fruits and vegetables.* Fruits contain essential nutrients that are under-consumed, including vitamin C, dietary fiber, and potassium, as diets rich in potassium help maintain healthy blood pressure. Most fruits are naturally low in fat, sodium, and calories. The AHA recommends adults eat four to five servings of fruits per day. You can add fruits to your diet by mixing sliced or frozen fruits with yoghurt or cereal. Or make fruit smoothies by blending fresh or frozen fruits, fruit juice, and yoghurt, or add dried or fresh fruit to oatmeal and waffles. Make sure to have a bowl of fruit where you can see and reach it on your desk at work or the kitchen counter. Vegetables also provide vital nutrients for the maintenance of your body. You can always add extra vegetables such as spinach, kale, and carrots to pasta sauces and soups. Add lots of vegetables when making a sandwich.

2. *Eat more fish.* Fish is a good source of protein and contains other vitamins and minerals. Compared to meat, fish has usually considered a healthier option due to its omega-3 fats content, which is good for the growth of the brain and protection from cancer and cardiovascular disease. The AHA recommends eating two servings of fish (especially oily fish) each week. A serving is 3.5 ounces of cooked fish or about three-quarters of a cup of flaked fish. Oily fishes have oil in their tissue and belly that

contains omega-3 fatty acids. Examples of oily fishes include tuna, herring, mackerel, sardines, and trout. Non-oily fish includes skate, haddock, catfish, and cod.

3. *Eat more high-fiber foods.* Foods like avocados, apples, broccoli, beans, and whole grains help maintain bowel health. It increases the weight and size of your stool and softens it. Fiber-rich foods help to solidify the stool because it absorbs water and adds bulk to stool. The AHA recommends that the daily value of fiber should be twenty-five gram per day on a 2000 calories diet for adults. Children between ages one and eighteen should eat fourteen to thirteen grams of fiber per day as the average American eats about sixteen grams of fiber per day.

4. *Reduce the intake of saturated fats.* Fats are vital in our diet as they help in reproduction. They absorb vitamin A, D, E, and K; and they also keep our body warm, but too much isn't right. There are two main types of fats you should be aware of: saturated and unsaturated. Saturated fats are bad fats as they stimulate the liver to produce more unhealthy low-density lipoprotein (LDLs). In contrast, unsaturated fats instigate the liver to produce healthy high-density lipoprotein (HLDs). Saturated fats are rife in many packaged foods, which can damage the liver. Children should have less saturated fat than adults, but a low-fat diet is not advisable for children under the age of five. Foods that contain saturated fats are butter, lard, sausages, fatty cuts of meat and cakes. A diet that contains unsaturated fats includes: olive and olive oil, oily fish, avocado and avocado oil, peanut and peanut butter, vegetable oils, almonds, and cashews.

5. *Eat less salt.* Consuming much salt has been proven to raise blood pressure, leading to various illnesses such as stroke and heart disease. About three-quarters of the salt you eat is already in the food you buy, such as breakfast cereals, bread, and soups. Adults and children aged eleven and over are advised to eat no more than six grams of salt (that's about a teaspoon) a day. Younger children should eat less. Salt contains sodium that the body uses to maintain fluid levels. A balance of sodium is necessary for the health of the heart, liver, and kidney. Too little sodium

in the body can lead to hyponatremia, confusion, muscle twitches, and dizziness. Most Americans take in too much salt, and seventy-five percent of it is hidden in processed and packaged food. The American Heart Association (AHA) recommends an intake of no more than 2,300 milligrams a day (that's about a teaspoon) and a limit of no more than 1,500 milligrams per day for most adults.

6. *Reduce your sugar intake.* Sugars are necessary for the production of energy in the body. Excess consumption of sugar through what you eat and drink increases the risk of obesity and tooth decay. Many packaged foods and drinks contain high amounts of free sugars. Free sugars are what we call any sugars added to foods by the manufacturer, cook, consumer, or found naturally in honey, syrups, and fruit juices. Sugars found in fruits and milk is more recommended for you to consume. Foods that contain free sugar include: biscuits, sugary drinks, sugary cereal, alcohol, chocolates, and sweets. Men should consume a maximum of nine teaspoons of sugar (thirty-six grams) per day, while women should consume about six teaspoons (twenty-five grams) per day.

The importance of physical activity as part of nutrition and health can't be overstated. Physical inactivity is already a significant global health risk. It is rife in both developed and developing countries, particularly among urban cities. Physical activity helps with energy expenditure, which is the primary cause of obesity and other obesity-related illness that leads to energy balance and weight control. The beneficial effect of physical activity on the body includes:

- It reduces the risk of chronic disease.
- It strengthens the muscles and bones.
- It lowers blood pressure.
- It improves blood circulation.
- It enhances memory.
- It reduces excess weight.

Here are some of the things you can do to build exercises into your day:

- Go for a walk at lunch.
- Use the stairs rather than the elevator or escalator.
- Dance around your home just for fun.
- Before going to work, try jugging or do a few sets of push-ups, burpees, or squats.
- Stretch your body often.
- Walk or ride a bike to your destination whenever possible.
- If you want to talk to your coworker, walk to their desk instead of sending emails or text.

Healthy diets and physical activity are essential to living a healthy lifestyle. The amount of energy you consume each day with the level of physical activity exhausted is the critical determinant of chronic nutrition disease. To maintain a healthy life, always remember to:

- Eat fruits and vegetables.
- Eat less fatty diets (especially food high in saturated fats or Trans fats).
- Consume food with less salt.
- And practice exercising that takes enough of your stored energy.

II

Part Two

LEADERSHIP and BUSINESS

Thank you for reading this far. Before you turn to the next chapter, I'd love to let you know that it would mean the world to me if you could leave an honest review on Amazon, Bookbub, or Goodreads of what you've read so far. A line or two is just enough and you could update the review when you've completed the book.

5

Principle #5: Socialize And Bond With People

Socializing is more positive than being alone. That's why meetings are so popular. — Mihaly Csikszentmihalyi

When I was a child, I would go out often to play with my friends. My friends and I would laugh together, buy the same biscuits, and sometimes cry together. Whenever my friend and I play sports, we would always make sure to be on the same team. Having friends around made me feel safe, happy, and comfortable. Humans are social beings with the desire to socialize and bond with others. Here's was what Brad, age 17, said about forming a relationship with his friends and family:

My peer group wants to make a difference. We are all doing well at school, and we want to keep it that way. We know there are bad things out there, and we want to help each other make the right decisions. My friends are like family to me, and we all look out for each other. It's what keeps me calm because I need them to support me when I need help. I'm there for them when they need me to. It's cool, and it works.

Forming relationships with people is beneficial to us as it allows for the growth of business and of human (especially children). We aren't wired to be alone or isolated from people. That could have meant death to our primordial ancestors, or loneliness, or depression. Without social relationships, the genus "homo" wouldn't have existed today. Developing good mental health and surviving depends on how much we relate to people, whether the right way or wrong. The essence of forming a social relationship with others is to achieve more than what we can by ourselves and to be safe.

Here is an interesting story that helps illustrate the importance of socializing:

Once upon a time, there lived a little boy. He was still a baby and didn't know any words except "mama" and "papa." But the boy's hands, feet, and eyes already knew how to speak. And one night, when the boy was lying in his crib, they started arguing about who is more important. "We're more important," the eyes claimed. "Without us, the feet wouldn't know where to go, and hands wouldn't know what to take." "No, we're more important!" the hands argued. "Sure, the eyes can see, but we're the ones playing with toys."

"You're both wrong; we are more important!" the feet shouted. "We're the ones that run to the toys in the first place." This argument was overheard by a magical elf that lived on a bookshelf full of fairy tales, next to the boy's crib. "All of you are very silly," he said. "Don't you realize that you are all helpless on your own? But together, you make up one body, agile and strong. And you're only important if you work together so that the boy can run, play, and look at the world. You have been entrusted with an important task: to protect the boy and help him. And here you are arguing with each other!

When the hands, the feet, and the eyes heard the elf's words, they became ashamed. They realized that they are all essential to the boy, and that made them happy. And they never argue anymore, but became friends and always worked together. And the baby grew up and became a happy and cheerful boy. Wherever there is harmony and friendship, growth and success do fall in.

How Socialization Affects Us: Adults and Children

In the old days, our primordial ancestors needed each other's support to survive, raise the children, and forage for food; not having a social group, just as it is in the animal kingdom, could mean starvation or death. When hominids wanted to forage or hunt for meat, they relied on the support of each other and the skills of each other to have a higher chance of surviving a predator attack and bringing food back home. Because being social has been an essential tool for our ancestors' survival, this trait has been genetically passed down for millions of years. Our need for being social can be a determining factor for our lust for interacting through social media, gossiping, and watching other's social interactions on reality TV shows. The evolutionary need to socialize and interact with people has become the cause of social pain that leads to depression and loneliness.

The importance of interacting with people is so strong that when we are isolated or feel rejected, we experience social pains and the brain begins to hurt just the same way our body feels physical pain. The need for children to socialize and interact with others is even more critical as it helps in cognitive development: thinking, reasoning, learning, and perception. Just as it is vital to eat, drink, and breathe, socializing is essential in brain circuitry development. For the growth of our neurons, we need other people's love, support, and interaction to survive and thrive. Children develop these abilities through the people they interact with. Putting children in an environment with other children, such as preschool or childcare, allows them to learn the skills to share with others, set boundaries, solve problems, and empathize with others as they recognize when their friends are sad or happy.

Children will eventually use these skills at home with their parents, siblings, and even pets. As we socialize with others, we pick up social cues that let us know what behaviours or reactions are appropriate and which ones aren't and the consequences of our actions. A California study published by the American Journal of Public Health suggests that social support networks may positively influence cognition and a protective association with dementia among other people. People who have no social friends have more than two times an increase in the risk of being cognitively impaired compared to those who have five or six social friends. People who find it difficult to build social ties and with people, even strangers, have a higher risk of developing mental and physical health problems—they can become lonely, stressed, and depressed.

"We've known for a long time that social skills are associated with mental health problems like depression and anxiety," Segrin said, the head of the UA Department of Communication. "But we've not known definitely that social skills were also predictive of poorer physical health. Two variables—loneliness and stress—appear to be the glue that binds poor social skills to health. Individuals with poor social skills have high levels of stress and loneliness in their lives." Segrin further said, "One of the problems with possessing poor social skills is lack of social awareness, so even if they're not getting the date, they're not getting the job, they're getting into arguments with co-workers or their spouse, they don't see themselves as the problem. They are walking around with this health risk factor, and they are not even aware of it."

Below are some of the negative consequences of not socializing with others affects mental and physical health.

1. *Depression.* Depression is one of the leading contributing factors to someone with poor social skills as they become isolated or alone. Because of our evolutionary need for socializing, studies have shown that people with fewer to none social ties have a substantial risk of being depressed. To avoid these from happening, experts recommend becoming more open to people, calling a long time friend, laughing with others, attending seminars or events with huge gatherings where you can interact with others, talking to your colleagues, and having fun with people.

2. *Loss of reality.* According to Emily Moyer-Guse, PhD, assistant professor of communication at Ohio State University in Columbus, in an interview with Huffington Post, people with poor social skills often spend most of their time on video games, binge watch TV shows or movies. They come to an end and become depressed due to the perceived loss of reality. Low

social skills can make you reduce your understanding of people, which leads you to express your emotions wrongly and blame others for your fault.

3. *It lowers self-esteem.* The loss of interaction with others reduces your self-confidence as you might begin to see people as a threat to you. That can allow you to become less comfortable associating and mingling with people.

4. *It decreases the ability to learn.* Just as children learn specific skills such as thinking, reasoning, solving a problem from their parents and friends, adults who are unable to associate with people have reduced mental capacity to learn new tasks to communicate well and solve complex problems.

5. *Decreased sense of empathy.* People with poor social skills have a reduced sense of understanding. They aren't able to attain social cues and understand human emotion because of isolation or less interaction with people. By isolating yourself, you're changing your brain's neurological circuitry and may hinder your ability to feel and express love to others.

6. *It shortens life longevity.* By making an effort to participate in social activities, the risk of depression, stress, anxiety, and loneliness reduces, which increases the quality of life. Adults who are not socially active have a higher risk of dementia, high stress, and loneliness, which can affect their immune system, mental and physical health.

The Negative Effect of Socializing

There are always two sides to a coin. Socializing has benefits. But it also has its downside (if not handled appropriately). Our brain is the most critical organ in the body. The brain alone consumes more energy than any other part of the body. Everything we do, from eating, walking, thinking, laughing, crying, loving, and being happy, is directed and controlled by the brain. Because your thoughts control your whole life, it is essential to feed your brain with the right information.

Our body reflects what we eat. If you consume high-calorie food, you are going to gain weight. If you consume too many sugary and starchy foods, you are most likely to develop dental problems. If you eat lots of fruits and vegetables, you will have healthier skin and a strong body. Physical stamina, a more robust immune system, body size, dental hygiene, and even how long we live are strictly related to what we eat. That's why every year, we spend millions of dollars on various dietary supplements to keep our bodies healthy.

Like our body, the mind reflects what is fed into it. Mind food is the information or stories we pick up from people and our environment. Mind food such as gossip, negative talk, and other forms of information belittles your thinking and influences you negatively. Positive self-talk, cheerful people, and other positive things make you feel more energetic and influence you positively.

Mind food is gotten from our environment—the people, culture, ideology, and things that can influence your conscious and subconscious thoughts. The people we associate with and learn from feed our minds, which means that our environment determines our attitudes, habits, and personalities. There is a famous saying: A child doesn't do what the parents want him/her to do, but a child does what the parent does. You are a mirror of the people you associate with.

In his book The Magic of Thinking Big, Dr. Schwartz asked these questions: Have you ever thought what kind of person you would be had you been reared in a different country? What types of food would you prefer? Would your clothing preferences be the same? What sort of entertainment would you like the most? What would your religion be?

If I am to predict the answer, I would say there would be a difference in the way we live. The culture of Kenyans is different from that of the Spanish people. China's religion is different from that of Americans. The marriage preparation of Mexicans is different from that of the Japanese. The food of Malaysians is different from the menu of Nigerians. Our actions, being the mirror of our outside world, means changing our world also changes our actions, habits, and personality. Remember this: Environment shapes us; it makes us who we are.

You are the average of at least five people you associate yourself with. From the way you laugh, dress, walk, dance, listen to music, and even talk, these are all influenced by the people you associate with and see on TV. If you hate reading, analyze the people you spend your time with, and you will notice a familiar pattern. A prolonged association with negative thinkers and doers makes you act like them. Continuous association with drug addicts would make you become one. However, there is a positive side to this. If you become aware of your close contact and hang around with positive people, this would influence you and give you the power to become the person you need, just by changing the people you associate with.

Close contact with big believers and big thinkers raises your level of thinking; close contact with optimistic people makes us confident. When you change friends, location, jobs, and foods, your mind changes as well. The individual you are right now is almost entirely not going to be the same individual you'll be five, ten, fifteen years from now. Your future self depends on your future environment. To change yourself, you have to change your environment. Make sure to vet the people and information you allow into your life as it can have a tremendous impact on how your life would turn out to be. Here are a few numbers of people you should avoid.

1. People who mess with your head.
2. People who intentionally and repeatedly do and say things that they know upset you.
3. People who don't want you or choose to grow.
4. People who expect you to prioritize them but refuse to prioritize you.
5. People who can't and won't apologize sincerely.
6. People who act like victims when confronted with their abusive behaviour.
7. Pessimistic people.
8. People who complain a lot and never take responsibility.
9. People who love to gossip.

To achieve and become successful, you have to abstain from negative people as they can slow down your momentum to achieve great things. Below are some tips from successful executives on how to stop negative people from getting in your way.

1. *Audit the five people in your social ties.* Gary Vaynerchuck, founder and CEO of VaynerMedia, and NYT- bestselling author, said:

Negative loser energy is a drag. Reflect on how you feel after hanging out with each of the closet people in your circle, after taking stock, audit accordingly. You may need to find new friends, people who are fired up and ready to win. You might even need to break up with your partner. Letting go is scary, but do you want to know the single most frightening thing of all time? Regret. Don't let loyalty trump your happiness.

2. *Consider why you're attracting negativity.* Roy McDonald, founder, and CEO of OneLife, said:

Whom we attract often reflects our behaviour. When encountering negative people, first consider why you're attracting their energy. To stop attracting negativity, you may have to give up some previous judgment. So ask yourself, "What is it about their negativity that frightens me so much?"

3. *Reflect before deciding.* Tom Shieh, CEO of Crimcheck, said:

It's easy to label others who don't share our attitude, perspective, or behaviour as "toxic" or "negative." Before cutting these "negative" people off, evaluate why their action triggers such intense emotions. And remember

- Removing fat doesn't create muscle,
- removing poverty doesn't create riches,
- removing coldness doesn't create heat,
- removing doubt doesn't create faith,
- removing darkness doesn't produce light,
- removing fear doesn't create courage,
- removing negativity doesn't create positivity.

4. *Explain your mission.* Tim Draper, legendary VC, founder of Draper Associations and DFJ, said:

All people have potential. I've turned negative people positive by explaining the mission, taking people through my thinking, and giving them my confidence that they can accomplish what I have in mind. When people understand the ultimate purpose of a task, activity, or goal and know it's achievable, they are more likely to work for it.

5. *Set rules.* Peter Hernandez, president of brokerage (California) at Douglas Elliman, cofounder of Teles Properties, said:

We tolerate negative people way too much, both professionally and socially. Instead, I follow these rules: One, avoid people who are cynical and critical. Two, don't waste time trying to fix them. Three, focus on people who love and support you. Four, be selective about who you let in. Five, part ways quickly and cleanly; don't get sucked back in. Six, remember Jim Rohn's quote: "You are the average of the five people you spend the most time with."

6. *Let negativity empower you.* Michael Johnson "The Mojo Master," speaker and mindset coach for professional athletes and elite entrepreneurs, said:

Negative people aren't always a problem. Sometimes, they can empower you to do something extraordinary, push harder, or inspire you to find your mojo. Some of my greatest achievements came because someone doubted me or tried to kick me down. I ask myself, "Is this person empowering or disempowering me?" I examine the benefits of their criticism. Usually, I'm being taught something myself to achieve more and be happier. If someone becomes negative and disempowering through their actions or consistent doubts, I slowly remove myself but never try to change them. It only creates resistance and resentment.

7. *Cut ties with yourself.* Mark Divine, retired US Navy SEAL commander, founder of SEALFIT, said:

The most crucial negative person to cut ties with is yourself. In Navy SEAL training, negativity surrounded me day in and day out. Some of it was orchestrated by our instructors to bring us down, but more came from my teammates fighting their conditioning and fear. You can't run from negative people, especially if they're essential in our life (such as family or work peers). The only thing you can do is learn to control your thoughts, emotions, and attitude while blocking any negative stories. It takes practice but is a crucial life skill to change everything for the better.

Connect with people and associate with friends. Design the environment you want and let it build you to become the individual you desire.

Working as a Team

Socializing is also essential to foster productivity at work and in personal relationships. It allows for better teamwork. Teamwork is an indispensable element for your own life, employment, and how you can focus and build new things. Cooperation is the combined and collaborative effort of a group to achieve a common goal or complete a task efficiently and effectively. Successful businesses like Starbucks, Pixar, and Apple rely on effective teamwork to succeed in their business. Collaboration isn't just crucial to the sports team, big corporation, military, but also to our relationships and schools. When you are in a relationship, consider your partner's opinion as well before making a decision that could affect both of you. Being part of a team involves sacrifices, selflessness, and perseverance.

A clear example of teamwork is the Apollo 11 mission in 1969. While many people recognized the three astronauts—Michael Collins, Buzz Aldrin and Neil Armstrong—that went for the mission; most remember only Armstrong and the famous one-liner he said upon being the first person to set foot on the moon: "That's one small step for a man, one giant leap for mankind." However, before the success of the historic mission are years of research and teams of hard-working people. Mission planners worked for two years before the launch, analyzing and studying the moon surface using satellite photographs to discern the best site for a lunar landing.

According to NASA, there were about 400,000 people who participated in making the lunar landing possible. It included teams of scientists, technicians, and engineers, many of who hadn't worked in aerospace before. The communication and connection that was involved between all groups allowed for a more cohesive team, which gave birth to the monumental success of the mission.

Good teamwork allows for more exceptional communication and cooperation between team members. When working together, it is critical to communicate effectively with one another to solve problems, complete tasks, develop creative ideas, and resolve conflict. It can be challenging to be a team player at work or in your relationships, but it is a skill that you can learn and improve. Improving teamwork can be done on an individual and group level, and a professional can help you hone and become more aware of your ability to work as a team. Here are some of the teamwork skills that are important to have to become a better teammate at work or at home.

1. *Conflict management.* Conflict is an inevitable situation that would occur in any group of people working together. The ability to resolve a conflict between team members is an essential skill of teamwork. When conflicts or verbal disputes do happen, which could often occur among team members, you need to settle disputes with your members and make sure everyone is happy with the team's decisions.

2. *Listening.* Listening is an important skill not just in teamwork, but it's also necessary to maintain a stable relationship. People who listen more than they speak tend to understand the other person's situation better. You must be able to listen to your peers' ideas and concerns to be an active and productive team member. Communicating with your peers by asking questions to demonstrate interests, clarification, and using nonverbal cues proves to your team that you care and are concerned about their opinions and ideas. There is a famous saying: when you speak, you are giving out information you already know. But when you listen, you are receiving new information. So do more listening and less of speaking.

3. *Respect.* Every healthy relationship and success of a big corporation relies on the connection each team member has for each other. No one ever wants to work or live with someone disrespectful. Showing respect by calling a person's name correctly or allowing a person to speak when communicating their ideas or concerns enables them to be more overt to your questions and feel respected.

4. *Communication.* Being able to articulate your thoughts with the team is essential, and it's one of the vital skills employers seek out from

employees. You should be able to convey your information via email, phone, and in person. Both verbal and nonverbal communication (i.e., eye contact, body movement, posture, facial expression, and tonality) are essential skills you should use when working.

5. *Give and receive feedback.* A good team player should give the team feedback, even if the input seems unpleasant to hear. You should also be able to collect opinions and ideas from your group members that might involve your poor performance, an opposing view to yours, or how poor your input to the group's growth has been. A person who understands and utilizes the feedback given is a leader who grows both himself and the team as a whole.

6. *Practice appreciation.* Nobody wants to feel unimportant or taken for granted. Everyone wants to be appreciated or praised. We crave for it. In a company or organization that doesn't value effort, we won't enjoy the job, and hence, we won't work at our best.

Whether you are in a relationship with your spouse, friends, or boyfriend/-girlfriend, there is no doubt that teamwork brings people closer together. A team that has gone through lots of trials and adversities and tackled severe problems together, within time, creates a special bond that brings them both closer together, on and off work. Research has also shown that individuals who work within a team that receives adequate support from the supervisors and team members have an increase in job satisfaction. It is essential to have cooperation in the workplace so that everyone can be more productive, less stressed, and relish their workdays.

Teamwork lightens the burden we carry alone. If not for collaboration, there would have been more stressed people in the community, fewer innovations, and low creativity. When you work together as a team, no one bears the responsibility of handling everything on their own. Teamwork is also essential in the home so that no one gets burned out by the stress of taking care of the children, tidying the house, and paying the bills.

"I have three children for John," Sarah said to me. "I work in a job that is stressful and requires most of my time. Mostly after coming back from work, before I could have time to rest, I would make sure to prepare meals for the children and John. I would assist with the children's assignment and make sure that it was done before the next day.

"When the laundry is full, I would be the one to do the laundry, since John doesn't even know how to operate the laundry machine. Sometimes, when he does come back from work, he often sits on the couch with his body smelling of smoke and stains of mechanical oil on his shoes and some parts of his body since he works at the mechanical department of a weaving factory. After sitting on the couch, before going to shower, he puts on the TV to watch his favourite series, and then requests his food."

"He treats me like I'm his maid," Sarah said painfully.

"The only help my husband majorly does," she said, "is to mow the lawn and clear the grass. That's all!"

"Is that so?" I asked bewildered.

"Not quite long," she continued, "I became frustrated. I felt used and unappreciated and was left alone doing all the tedious work in the house. I expressed my thoughts to John and suggested we go for counselling. He was resistant at first, but he later acquiesced. A month later, we went to meet with a counsellor. The counsellor spoke a lot of things and threw us a few questions to verify where the problem was coming from.

"To John's surprise, the counsellor was able to deduce that the cause of the relationship's friction was because of John's unappreciative and unsupportive attitude towards me."

"John was perplexed," Sarah said.

"How can this be?" John asked in bewilderment.

"I go to work five days a week," John continued his remark, "spending hours working my face off. And don't forget, I also help pay the bills at home."

"I don't dispute that," Sarah responded with a calm tone.

But the counsellor also responded, "John, you claim to be very busy, which is true; however, your wife also has a lot of work on her plate. If I am not mistaken, from what I have gathered, Sarah also works five days a week; she helps get the laundry done, takes care of the children, cleans the house, and cooks the meal for the family."

"Isn't that too much work for just one person?" the counsellor asked.

John took a second to gather his thought. "I guess so," he replied with a guilty voice.

"That day, John became aware of his faults and promised to make changes," Sarah said. "Before leaving, the counsellor gave us some tasks we both should do while we get home. During the first week, there wasn't a lot of changes from him, but I didn't rush him because I knew it would take some time to quit his harmful habit. However, about two to three weeks later, he learned how to operate the laundry machine, and he also learned how to cook certain meals that he could prepare for the family during weekends.

"I was glad when I saw these changes in him. But that wasn't all. He also chose to help me with some of the chores at home, like cleaning the electronics and arranging the bedroom and the children's room. And he also increased the number of 'thank you,' he says to me."

"This greatly brought me joy," Sarah spoke with smiles, "and made me a pleased wife and mother."

The point is apparent. Make it a rule to let others know you appreciate what they do for you. Remarks like, "I don't know what I would do without you." "Thank you for yesterday," would go a long way in making the other person feel much better and perform better—practice appreciation with honest, personalized compliments. Give a warm, sincere smile. Smiles lets others know that you notice their efforts and feel kindly towards them. A team that appreciates each other's energy is a team that thrives and succeeds.

Handling Difficult People

Have you ever come across someone who frustrates you so much that you begin to vent your anger or just scream out loud? We've all been there. The truth is, you can't reason with an unreasonable person, and a group of more than four individuals has a high probability of having a difficult person (or black sheep) among the group. Over the years, I've encountered my fair share of difficult people: people who don't show up for meetings, people who don't complete their work as promised, people who believe vehemently in their views and refuse to collaborate, and people who fail to take responsibility for their poor decisions. It is not uncommon for a family or friend of four or more to likely have someone who would often make you frustrated, angry, and lose your sanity.

There are times when difficulties were getting a consensus in the team because everyone was so firm on their views. There are times when I'd think, "Why are these people so difficult?" "These people are so irresponsible!" Or "I don't ever want to work with this group of individuals again!" A common question that most people would ask is, "Can't I work with another team?" But the fact is that difficult people are all around us—they are in our homes, workplace, churches, military, and schools. So understanding techniques on how to deal with such people is the only way for you not to lose your sanity each day.

1. *Be calm.* We've all heard, at some point, someone telling us to "be calm" when we go wild. Losing your temper and flaring out at the other person isn't the best way to get him/her to work with you. No one likes to be shouted at; it only increases the tension between both parties. Someone who protrudes calmness and equanimity is seen as being in control, centered, and more respectable. When the person you are having a confrontation with sees that you are calm despite whatever he/she does, you will begin to get their utmost attention. And if being peaceful isn't enough to quell the argument, try the next step.

2. *Understand the person's intention.* There is an old belief that: people don't just do anything without a reason. When you notice a person acting in such a way to you, but different from others, try to understand their underlying motive. Try to ask yourself and understand: what is making this person act in this manner? What is stopping him/her from cooperating with me? How can I help to meet his/her needs and resolve the situation? Understanding the motives of a person is an important step in de-escalating a case.

3. *Let the person know where you are coming from.* One thing that has worked

for me is to let the person know my intentions behind what I am doing. Sometimes, the reason why people are resistant to you is that they see you for who you are not. They think you will cheat on them or backstab them based on their experience with another person. Articulating the real intentions behind your actions lets them understand that you mean no harm, but the best for them. That would enable him/her to break the barrier that allows for better collaboration.

4. *Build a rapport.* With all the computers, emails, and messaging systems, work can sometimes turn into a mechanical process. Re-instil the human connection by relating with your colleagues on a personal level. During breaks or closing periods, set out a date with them. Go to lunches or dinner, play sports together, or visit their home and spend time with their family. Get to know them as people and not just colleagues. This kind of gesture would be interpreted to them as a sign of true friendship that surpasses the camaraderie of just being work buddies. It builds trust, which would go a long way in your work.

5. *Ignore.* If you've already tried everything above and done all you can do to repair the relationship, but the person isn't still receptive, the best way might be to ignore it. Some people will choose not to reconcile with you, no matter what. All you need to do is continue with your daily task and connect with the person only if necessary.

6. *Report to a higher authority for resolution.* When all else fails, report to your manager. It is considered the trump card and shouldn't be used unless you've completely exhausted your means. There is a reason why we have police to report to when things get out of hands. Be careful not to exercise this option all the time as you wouldn't want your manager to think that you are incapable of handling your problems. When you've tried all you can do to deescalate the situation, report to or involve someone that's of higher power or authority that may handle the situation better.

We all need people to grow our mental abilities; we need people to feel great, learn new skills, and survive. Understanding what types of people are allowed in your social circle is an essential determinant of your success. Always try to connect yourself with people and be a team player. Appreciate those that help you in your life and don't make them feel they're being used or taken for granted. You can't survive alone, even in our technological world. So socialize with long time buddies, call a family member, do things you haven't done or are too afraid to do—sky jump, go to a video game event, or ride an insane roller coaster. And remember: Your diet isn't just what you put into your body; it's also what you put into your mind. Feed yourself with the right mind food. The best way to change your life is to: first, be aware that you need change. Second, analyze your environment, vet your social circle, assess the information you consume, and pinpoint those mind foods that negatively influence you and drain your energy and time. Third, make changes—take action!

6

Principle #6: Don't Work Alone

One is too small a number to achieve greatness. No accomplishment of real value has ever been achieved by a human being working alone. —
John C. Maxwell.

Steve Jobs started his first business with Steve Wozniak, a very close high school friend and an electronic engineer. In 1971, Wozniak and Jobs designed the "Blue box," a device for phreaking (hacking into the telephone network without paying for long-distance calls) that they began selling to students. Wozniak and Jobs were members of the Homebrew Computer Club, where they quickly became enamoured with kit computers and left the Blue Box behind. The next product they made and sold was the Apple I, which was just a motherboard without a monitor and keyboard. The customers needed to add their monitor and keyboard to make use of it. The production of Apple I helped the hobbyist get enough capital to build the Apple II in 1977. Apple II made the company. Wozniak, being an exceptional engineer, built both these computers, and Jobs handled the marketing and sales aspect of the business. Jobs and Wozniak created enough interest in their new product to attract venture capital. It meant their company, Apple, was officially incorporated in 1976.

There is no doubt that each one of us is blessed with exceptional abilities to achieve a whole lot all by ourselves. If we focus and dare our minds to think bigger, we can achieve bigger. But there is a misconception in the public's view. When most people see top executives and founders who manage successful companies like Apple, Microsoft, and Alibaba, most think that these people achieve these great feats alone. That couldn't be further from the truth.

Before Steve Jobs met Steve Wozniak, he had nothing. He was a poor, adopted child. Wozniak, also, didn't have much. Wozniak was just a guy that loved electronics. When Job met Wozniak, he was fascinated by how skilled Wozniak was in electronics. Although Jobs knew about electronics, Wozniak was on a different level compared to him. The love they both shared for their work bonded them together, which later led them to build the world's first company to achieve $1 trillion market capitalization.

Without the expertise and relationship, both had, each person wouldn't have achieved what they both made. To create a fortune 500 company, remarkable technology, and great scientific discoveries, you'll need to collaborate with others. An ample number of people have been convinced that to create a successful brand or product, we can do that all by ourselves—that you don't need anyone's help. That is the fastest way to dig your way to failure. In our competitive age, everyone is trying to be the first to create the latest technology, make discoveries, or find a vaccine for a new virus; the winners are those who have chosen to work together.

In schools, we are always taught to do things ourselves, not ask anyone for tips or answers. We have been told that asking for help is cheating. The teacher would say, "If you ask for help from your classmate, it means you are dumb." However, in the real world, that's not the case. Let's look at two different people who took different approaches to achieve their ambitions. The first took the "school" approach; the second person took the "collaborative" approach.

BLAKE

Blake is a graduate student from a well-known institution. Before being admitted to college, he always had the idea of creating the next big social media service. He was fascinated with software and technology. At the age of twelve, his father bought him a computer that he used to learn to program. He would spend most of his time online doing research and learning about coding languages. When he was admitted to college, it was evident to his parents and friends that he would study software development. After spending five years in college and learning all he thought he needed to make an excellent social app, he began building the app.

Blake was a smart student at college—a straight-A student. He took the advice of his lecturer, "Always do things yourself," "Don't ask for help; you have the internet," "You've got to do things alone for you to be really smart " He took all of this advice to heart. He always thought of his app as being the next big thing that would shake the world and get everyone talking and excited. He learned about the various programming languages—Php, Java, C++, and Javascript—he needed to build his app. After months of intense focus and determination, Blake finished his app. But he noticed a problem. The user interface and user experience (UI/UX) was appalling. Blake wasn't great at this since it wasn't his speciality. Rather than seeking out people who have years of experience in UI/UX, he decided to take his lecturer's advice: "Don't ask for help, you have the internet."

Blake went online and bought a course on UI/UX that made him spend an extra month learning the nooks and crannies of it, which significantly delayed his project. After fixing the UI/UX problem, the app still didn't look great. Since he couldn't be an expert by just watching a video and practising for a month, he was O.K. with the result. But Blake noticed another problem with his app—the design. Again, he held on to his lecturer's advice and decided to buy another course on the design. This made him spend about seven weeks more, learning and practising. The design he learned improved his app aesthetics, but again, it didn't look great, still. When he thought he had everything done, he decided to pitch his new app to investors. When he met the investors, his face exuded gladness, he was thrilled. He had always thought of reaching the point of pitching and displaying his app.

However, something was wrong again! The investors wanted to understand his vision and be as enthusiastic as he was, they just couldn't. Blake might be a good app creator or programmer, but he wasn't skilled in business and communication. Because he wasn't able to properly communicate his vision to the investors, they couldn't get on board. Blake got lots of NOs from different investors that later made him quit.

JOSIE

Josie, like Blake, is a graduate student from a well-known institution. Josie loves electronics, technology, and software. When she got admitted to college, she immediately associated herself with friends from different departments that she thought would be of great use for her social media app ambition. She wasn't a straight-A student and never thought it was necessary to be one. Although, like Blake, her lecturer often says words like: "Make sure to not seek for help and study on your own so you don't become dependent on others," "You have the internet; what else do you want?" But Josie never held on to that ideology when dealing with the real world.

Before graduation, she became close with a lot of friends from different department with different expertise. After graduation, Josie called some of her friends that she knew would play an essential part in creating her app beautifully and make it a global success. Josie held a meeting and invited them to her house, where she talked about the idea to them. Because she had a good relationship with them and some of them were quite conversant about her plan, they decided to help.

Her friends included people who had expertise in design, business analysis, UI/UX, product management, performance testing, and communication. Fortunately for Josie, she didn't have to pay them much because they knew each other, and they were pumped for the task. In less than five months, with intense focus, they were able to create the app she envisaged.

Before pitching their app to investors, they decided to share the app with people to use for a few weeks so they could gather their feedback and know what changes they need to make. After making the necessary changes, they were able to pitch their idea to investors. Unlike Blake, Josie surrounded herself with people who knew how to get investors interested in her views. After tossing her concept to a few investors, she got her YES. The capital allowed her and her team to get a proper office, more workers, and payment to continue developing the app until it became global.

Everyone is talented, creative, and ambitious to come up with ideas and produce impressive products, but you alone can't create mind-blowing results. We all need someone to collaborate with to make significant achievements. Like many of us, Blake's school ideology prevented him from associating with others, recognizing real talent in others, and realizing his dream. Working with like-minded people doesn't make you a loser or a failure; instead, it makes you a leader and a winner. The things you could achieve from a good team are far higher than what you could achieve alone.

Every successful person always has at least one person to thank for their success. It might be a school friend, your spouse, or your parents. It doesn't matter. In reality, a team of right players would always beat a single all-time champion player. In reality, Bruce Lee can never win against one hundred fighters. All successful businessmen and women don't play the game alone; they always have a team of experts—Steve Jobs and Steve Wozniak, Bill Gates and Steve Ballmer, Walt Disney and Roy Disney—just to name a few.

In every example of great leaders and products that have achieved remarkable results, there was always a person or a small group of people who knew how to make the vision a reality. For example, Josie gathered the right people who knew how to make her app the way she wanted it. Steve Job had Wozniak, who was good at making stuff. Jobs was an extraordinary visionary, with an intense and often combative management style, and Wozniak, on the other hand, was the genius who made the vision work. Working together with others speeds up and improves the results significantly. As discussed in chapter 5, socializing and associating with people was the only way to guarantee our ancestors' survival.

No one is an island of knowledge, and no one should try to know everything because: First, it is impossible for your brain to have all the information that possibly exists. There's only so much that our brain can remember and keep in the conscious mind. Second, it will cost you more time.

Having a team of people to work with shortens the time to complete tasks.

You don't have to work on your own. To experience a remarkable result, you have to work with great people. You must have the desire to create a capable team. An effective team involves people with diverse expertise and the ability to work fluently with each other to achieve a common goal or task. Each team member is vital as they play an essential role in the team's success; no one is less important.

Four primary characteristics are common to all successful businesses and groups. I call it the 4Cs of team success: clarity, competence, commitment, and consistency.

1. *Clarity.* Successful business or group must be able to clearly interpret the team members' vision, objectives, and values. A good leader must clearly state WHAT they need to achieve, HOW to achieve it, and WHEN it's to be completed. A sailor without a compass for direction will in no time be lost. A team without a clear sense of direction, of course, is a lost team. Each team member should be able to know where the business is heading, so they can be able to direct their effort to make that a reality. Each team member should know what the company's values and goals are and clearly understand what role and responsibility they have. When Jobs and Wozniak initially started their Blue Box and Apple I business, they both realized their responsibilities: Jobs was in charge of sales and marketing; Wozniak was in charge of production. Also, team members should be clear about the company's standard of excellence.

2. *Competence.* Companies that aim to succeed must have team members who don't only know what they're responsible for (their job), but they must also know how to get their job done. Josie understood the importance of competence. She knew that for her to have a chance of succeeding, she observed the need to have people that know how to do their work and produce the right result in the team. It's one thing to be clear about what to do; it's another thing to be able to do it. Competence gives team members the skill required to perform what is expected of them. It's not enough to have lots of people working on a project; they must be able to have the right behaviour and skills necessary to

produce results. Team members must operate at their best; they must be identified in their place of strength: the area where they excel most. Supposing Jobs and Wozniak were to change the roles they both played in the making of Apple Company; they probably wouldn't have had the success they achieved. George S. Patton once said, "Success demands a high level of logistical and organizational competence." If you don't have the right people in your team for the job, expect your business to get tanked.

3. *Commitment.* It's one thing to know what to do. It is one thing to be able to do it. It's yet another thing to do it wholeheartedly. Every task comes with its trials, but team members must be able to commit to the team's vision, goals, and objectives, as well as to one another. Nothing great ever comes easy. Only those who are committed to their vision and ideas achieve success. When people are driven by their commitments, they bring their zest to the task and complete their duty with excellence. Both Blake and Josie were committed to their vision, but as we've seen, commitment alone wasn't enough to achieve remarkable success. You also need consistency.

4. *Consistency.* This is a crucial factor for success. A wise man once said: "Without commitment, you'll never start; more importantly, without consistency, you will never finish." Whatever way you want to look at it, those words would always stand true. All high achievers have embedded consistent rituals in their day, which brings extraordinary success. It is not just enough to be committed to a goal or task, but you also have to take continuous steps and effort, be it rough or smooth, to reach the point of extraordinary achievement. Consistency is essential to the success of a business. For example, Apple Inc. must be consistent in its production of exceptional products because customers buy their product to expect the same kind of innovative products they've always been producing. If they stop innovating or making great products, even for a day, they will lose customers. If leaders aren't consistent with their vision, it can demoralize the employees and reduce the company's value. Know this: Success is the inevitable and predictable result of consistent

actions, rather than intensity.

Wilbur and Orville Wright were American inventors and pioneers of aviation. Their father, Milton Wright, was a bishop in the Church of the United Brethren in Christ. He would often buy them small toys. In 1878, he bought them a small model helicopter (made of cork, bamboo, paper, and powered by a rubber band to twirl its blades) for his boys. Fascinated by the toy and its mechanics, Wilbur and Orville would develop a lifelong love for aeronautics and flying.

Wilbur and Orville set to work, trying to figure out how to design wings for flight. They observed that birds angled their wings for balance and control, and tried to emulate this, developing a concept called "wing warping." When they added a moveable rudder, the Wright brothers got it right. Between 1899 and 1905, the Wright brothers conducted aeronautical research and experimentation that led to the first successful powered aeroplane in 1903. Wilbur flew their plane for 59 seconds, at 852 feet—an extraordinary achievement. Two years later, they made a practical flying aeroplane.

The moral of the story is: be clear, be competent; be committed; be consistent. And don't work alone.

Blind Spots in leadership and Business

Believe it or not, you have blind spots. I have blind spots, like everyone else. People who don't believe they have blind spots give themselves false impressions that they can see all things right before it happens—economic depression, economic boom, potential risk, or reward. But it is a simple fact that no one by themselves can see the complete picture of reality. Our life experience has shaped us to see things differently. Folks that have spent a considerable part of their life in a thug community would likely instil a thug attitude when they are grown.

People born with a silver spoon would probably not understand what it means to lack. People that have spent years in business would understand better how to run a sustainable business. Folks that have spent years in the music industry would appreciate a lot about music, but little to nothing about politics. The point is: you only know what you've opened yourself to. Blind spots are everywhere in your lives; from your behaviours to your relationships, and more. Others may notice what we are missing, but we may be oblivious to our actions because of the blind spots. A large number of us only see what we expect to see. When your mind is focused on one thing, it can turn a blind eye to the other things that might come your way. Thus, leaders cannot see the coming of an economic depression, the potential of significant loss, or the value of an emerging idea that doesn't fit within their current expectations.

The majority of companies and businesses have blind spots. Major companies have been taken out due to their blind spots. In 1998, Yahoo (a web services provider) refused to buy Google for only $1 million. In 2002, Yahoo realized their mistake and tried to buy Google—this time for $3 billion, but Google asked for $5 billion. Yahoo said, No! In 2008, Yahoo refused to be sold to Microsoft for $44.6 billion. In 2016, Yahoo was sold to Verizon for $4.6 billion.

When yahoo refused to acquire Google—twice, they were unable to see the strength of Google. When Yahoo refused to be sold to Microsoft, they were unable to see their imminent downfall. Sadly, Yahoo isn't the only company that was affected by the blind spot.

In 2000, Reed Hastings approached former Blockbuster CEO John Antioco and asked for $50 million to give away the company he founded—Netflix. Everyone from Blockbuster who was at the meeting must cringe when they think back on it now. Antioco, thinking that it was a "tiny niche business," ended the negotiation and didn't buy Netflix, which at the time was a DVD-by-mail rental service. He seemed to see it as a big joke. Now Netflix has a market capitalization of $187.3 billion, putting it just over Disney's $186.6 billion. You and I, just like Yahoo and Blockbuster, could have made the same mistake. No one is immune to blind spots, but we can limit it. It is almost impossible not to have blind spots in business, relationships, and behaviours. In organizations, it can be challenging to know all of your customers' minds and understand how they view and interact with your product. This is prevalent in the phone industry.

Major phone manufacturers are focusing mainly on the development of their cameras. Phones are coming out with better, sharper, and more cameras than ever before. But what if the customers don't need a better camera? What if we are satisfied with the camera's quality and quantity? What if what we need is a better battery life that would be enough to last through the day? As of the time of this written, most opulent phones have a battery capacity between 3500 – 4000 mAh. That can be improved since other phone manufacturers are doing so. What if what their customer wants is a cheaper phone that's also powerful enough to work? That can certainly happen if the phone manufacturers are not blind to see it.

Blind spots can significantly affect large companies; there are so many people and departments and conditions that we simply can't keep track of in all aspects of the business. We are so immersed in our product and corporate culture that it becomes hard for us to have a truly objective view of our company. When we prepare ourselves for certain events to occur, we sometimes get hit by something we didn't expect. When we work together with people of different backgrounds, behaviour, knowledge, and expertise, we are more likely to foresee the probability of something happening before it happens. We become more aware of the bigger picture. Events change faster than we would expect when we fail to see and prepare for it, which can be detrimental to a company's success.

For example, today, the printing business has undergone some changes as digital technology transform the need and use of printed materials. Newspapers, books, greeting cards, posters, and brochures are being replaced with digital technology. Those in the printing business are scrambling for ways to innovate, with many seeking to integrate to expand services and develop new profit centers vertically.

FedEx transformed how we ship packages. The U.S. postal services did not see it coming, but the business plan was also rejected when submitted in a college course. Blackberry was an outstanding phone that everybody wanted to use before the rise of the iPhone. Blackberry failed to innovate. They ignored the touchscreen-based technology, and Apple started to dominate the mobile phone market.

Here are some of the technologies or industries that are rapidly advancing or experiencing breakthroughs and can potentially disrupt the current economy:

- Virtual Reality (VR) and Augmented Reality (AR)
- Advanced robotics
- Artificial Intelligence (AI)
- Internet of Things (IoT)
- Renewable Energy
- 3D Printing
- Energy Storage
- Mobile Internet

How do organizations and business leaders avoid the effect of blind spots?

To change, you need to be aware of the need for change and be mindful of your environment. You need to be conscious that you have blind spots and then figure out what they are and how to get past them. By expanding your consciousness, you open yourself up to seeing more of what is there to see. For a company to avoid blind spots, it has to recognize and monitor trends in other industries, and their own, to ensure they understand the changes happening and how it might impact them. But identifying the latest trends in an industry is not enough to mitigate the blind spots. There are certain practices we need to adopt to reduce blind spots.

1. *Discourage groupthink.* Groupthink occurs when a group of individuals makes a unanimous decision without critical reasoning or evaluation of the consequences or alternatives. In a business, groupthink can cause both employees and managers to overlook potential problems in the pursuit of consensus thinking. Whenever you hear someone on your team begin with something like, "We all agree to...," "I believe everyone is on board with...," it could mean that your team has fallen into a

groupthink. Instead, promote speaking for one's self. Allow everyone to express their concerns and opinions. Tell people to speak for themselves. It creates an environment where thoughtful disagreement and counter views can be expressed without fear of reprisal. Dina Badie, an Assistant Professor of Politics and International Studies at Center College, argued that the invasion of Iraq by the United States was driven by groupthink. According to Badie, after 9/11, stress, promotional leadership, and intergroup conflict were the factors responsible for the shift in the U.S. administration's view on Saddam Hussien that eventually led to military action in Iraq.

2. *Cut down the hierarchy barrier*. Be open to ideas from your subordinates. Seek their feedback, opinions, and insight about an issue, no matter how silly it might be. Because people see things differently than you do, you are more likely to receive reasonable solutions from unexpected people. Ensure that you and other top management teams are available to any staff, even customers who want to be involved in the discussion or have a different suggestion to the matter being discussed. You may be surprised at the outcome.

3. *Shake it up*. Don't be afraid to change things a bit. Move out of your comfort zone by implementing activities that break the company's tradition. Create an environment that encourages people to ask questions, raise important issues, and challenge the status quo. When you notice that your company's path is becoming obsolete, don't be afraid to make changes even if it's a new one. Allow your employees to work on themselves (on projects that may not be related to your market or industry) and be creative. Most times, that is where a profound idea comes from.

Make sure to eliminate the idea of doing things alone. You alone can't see all of the challenges and opportunities of this world. Only those who embrace the support and knowledge of others truly make remarkable things happen.

Mentors

If you studied physics at school, then you've probably heard of Newton's Laws of Motion. It contains three laws, but we would address the first law. It states that: Every object remains in a state of rest unless acted upon by an external force. What the law means is, if you are a sloppy person, you would always remain sloppy unless acted upon by an external force (motivation). If you are well organized, you will forever remain organized unless you are moved by an external force (lousy circle of friends). Newton's first law of motion helps us understand why the rich continue to become rich, and the poor continue to grow poor. Unless a more potent outside force impacts you, you won't garner the momentum to change your state of sloppiness and low income. That is why we need mentors.

Having an experienced mentor is a life-changing experience and precious to your personal and professional development. A mentor is a friend or person who guides a less experienced person by building trust and modelling positive behaviours. Most youth organizations now recognize the importance of having a mentor. Approximately three million adult volunteers are involved in a formal, one-on-one mentoring relationship with young people; an increase of seventy-nine percent (500,000 mentors) since 2000. Consistent studies have shown that students who meet regularly with their mentors are fifty-two percent less likely than their peers to skip a day of school and thirty-two percent less likely to skip a class. Mentoring increases social acceptance, academic attitudes, and grades. For children who come from less than ideal circumstances, mentoring is vital for a positive youth outcome.

Urie Bronfenbrenner, a developmental psychologist, said, "development, it turns out, occurs through this process of progressively more complex exchange between a child and somebody else—especially somebody crazy about that child."

Everyone can and should have a mentor. They help to lead, direct, and comfort you during tumultuous times. When we look at people with great success—Bill Gates, Richard Branson, and Oprah Winfrey—we think they achieved their success based on talent, skill, or a genius mind. But we often fail to understand that they had several people who helped them along the way and helped direct and rush them to success.

Here are some of the famous mentors and mentees that you might know.

1. Barbara Walters mentored Oprah Winfrey. During an interview, Oprah told Babara Walters: "Had there not been you, there would never have been me."

2. Warren Buffett mentored Bill Gates. Bill Gates and the investor genius Warren Buffett met in 1991 and have been friends for almost twenty-nine years. Gates admits that he has turned to Buffett for advice on various subjects over the years and has often referred to Buffett as "One of a kind." Gates also greatly admires Buffett's "desire to teach things that are complex and put them in a simple form, so that people can understand and benefit from all his experience."

3. Sir Freddie Laker mentored Richard Branson. Richard Branson once said, "If you ask any successful business person, they will always say they have had a great mentor at some point along the road." Branson asked English Airline entrepreneur, Sir Freddie Laker, for guidance during his struggle to get Virgin Atlantic off the ground. Branson wrote in the British newspaper, the Sun: "It's always good to have a helping hand at the start. I wouldn't have got anywhere in the airline industry without the mentorship of Sir Freddie Laker."

4. Steve Job mentored Mark Zuckerberg. In an interview with American talk show host Charlie Rose, Mark Zuckerberg, co-founder of Facebook, talked about his inspiring mentor Steve Jobs: "He was amazing. I had a lot of questions for him." Zuckerberg described how Jobs gave him advice about building a team focused on building "high quality and good things." Both men wanted to change the lives of people. In a final farewell Facebook post to Jobs, Zuckerberg wrote: "Thanks for showing that what you build can change the world."

Contrary to what your thoughts might be, mentors can also learn from mentees. In an interview, Buffett said: "What I really must admire about Bill

is the view he has about what he should do with the wealth he's accumulated...
he knows he's a beneficiary of a terrific society." Great mentors are people
who enjoy learning and growing, even from their mentees. There are many
qualities a good mentor should have. Here are some.

1. *The mentor should be right for you.* There are many good people out there
   that you can pick as your mentor, but they must fit your style. Many
   people will try to manipulate and take advantage of you and your career;
   they would try to influence and develop you to their image rather than
   figuring out what your needs are. A good mentor will create a strategy
   that fits your needs, talent, and desires and push you towards a better
   you—not towards a clone of themselves.

2. *Mentors enjoy learning new things.* Good mentors understand that while
   they are experts, they can't possibly know everything. These are people
   that have books or digital forms of books with them anywhere they go,
   and they want to pass that desire on to everyone they meet. Warren
   Buffett spends five to six hours a day reading five newspapers and 500
   pages of corporate reports. Bill Gates reads fifty books a year. Mark
   Zuckerberg aimed to read at least one book every two weeks. Mark Cuban
   reads for more than three hours every day. Arthur Blank, a co-founder
   of Home Depot, reads two hours a day. Good mentors will be excited to
   share their knowledge with you and be willing to explore the possibility
   that you may know what they don't.

3. *Mentors should be enthusiastic about their role.* When you are looking for
   a mentor, make sure to pick the one with an enthusiastic personality.
   They need to be passionate and excited about the role. You should feel
   their sincerity in the way they present their desire to help you. Buffett is
   always willing and happy to share his knowledge with Gates and help
   him with specific problems. Good mentors should be ready to teach
   others and receive rewards, not in the form of materialistic items or
   money, but in seeing the people they helped become more successful
   than they are.

4. *Mentors should provide honest feedback.* Feedback is essential to the

growth of any person. Because of the blind spot we all have, people need input from other eyes to help us continue to improve in our goals and skill. The feedback should not demoralize you but should make you recognize your shortcomings and identify corrective actions you can take to progress.

Jim Rohn once spoke these words: My mentor said, "Let's go do it, not, you go do it." So, your mentor should work with you as you both learn, grow, and inspire each other.

7

Principle #7: Have It If You Want It

Victory is always possible for the person who refuses to stop fighting. —
Napoleon Hill.

It takes will and determination to chase a dream and succeed. A lot of folks
have given up on themselves and their goals. They've succumbed to their
inner voices, "I can't make it," "It's too hard," "I don't have what it takes,"
"I don't have the degree," "Who am I to become successful?" Or perhaps,
they've accepted the demoralizing talk their friends and society have said
to them. But you shouldn't listen to your inner negative-talk or from those
around you. You can succeed; if you put your mind to it. You don't have to go
to school, and you don't have to be a graduate to succeed. What you aspire
doesn't have to be comfortable to achieve, and everyone doesn't have to agree
with you or understand your dreams.

Most of the success achieved didn't come easy. Many successful people
didn't have much money to start with, and many people didn't believe in
them initially. You don't have to have rich parents for you to excel. Based
on 2018 data, according to a report published by Wealth-X, that analyzed
the world's wealthy population (those with a net worth of $30 million or
more). Of the 265,490 wealthy individuals, 67.7 percent were self-made,
while 23.7 percent had a combination of self-made and inherited wealth.

Only 8.5 percent of global high net-worth individuals had their wealth by inheritance. Certain traits are responsible for the increase in self-made millionaires and billionaires.

Focus

Always remember, your focus determines your reality. — George Lucas

Distraction is a common theme for everyone. Everyone gets distracted; some people more than others, but no one is immune. Bringing your attention back to what's essential and gaining focus is critical to getting things done effectively and efficiently. It doesn't matter how enthusiastic you are about a task; if you don't focus enough, you will screw things up and waste a lot of time; in the end, it's all about getting things done.

The importance of focus on personal and professional life can't be overstated. How you use your attention, moment to moment, dramatically determines what kind of person you become. Our minds and lives are shaped mainly by how we use them. All great products, inventions, and discoveries are made because of the focus and attention invested in them. According to Daniel Goleman, author of Emotional Intelligence, the link between focus and excellence is behind almost all our achievements. Your focus and concentration are great tools and skills that you should develop to the fullest to be more productive and to make things better, attain goals, and maintain a healthy relationship.

Distraction is the enemy of productivity. Without the ability to focus, you'll lose the ability to think creatively, reason, learn, solve problems, and make decisions. Without focus, you won't be able to concentrate on a task, which will make you less efficient and less effective. Focus is an important character to consider when recruiting people to work. Distraction doesn't allow for a productive result and reduces work quality; it only increases the time of completing a task.

A distracted mind produces poor results. A focused mind, on the other hand, produces excellent results. If you can't focus right, you won't think effectively. Many people's excuse for not producing great results is often, "I am too busy," "I have lots of work to do," but the main reason is that they are too distracted. Humans have created a world that makes it very easy to get distracted. Social media, TV, advertisements have distracted you from the most crucial thing—You! Focusing on activities and tasks that are important to you is essential for productive growth. A focused mind can complete tasks far quicker than a distracted mind.

It is essential to focus on one task and one task only. To set your attention on more than one task means lesser productivity. And don't think about multitasking. The chance of you having the ability to multitask is thin. Studies have shown that only two percent of people can multitask effectively. Ninety-eight percent of people who try to multitask, tend to impair their productivity more than help it. For those monotaskers like me, it's essential to focus on one task at a time for better quality work, at a quicker rate. Being focused means removing all distractions and giving your full undivided attention to a particular job.

The rise of the internet and TV shows has made it difficult for people to even think about what is important to them. It is difficult to think straight when you are living in a society that is never settled. Chaos is prevalent in many countries, communities, and at home, and it has shifted people's focus away from their goals to their security. The tension between countries are rising, crimes are increasing, the economy is heading into a depression, paychecks are reducing, the morbidity rate is on a high, politicians are stealing from the people, and the poor are robbing the poor. All of these unsettles the mind and shifts people's focus away from developing themselves to protecting themselves. That's why there has been an increase in firearm sales in America. In 2019, a survey found that around 37 percent of households in the US reported owning one or more firearms. This makes the US the most heavily armed civilian population in the world.

There is a rise in advertisements and marketing messages, as so many people are trying to get our attention to buy their products. It is difficult to get away from all these distractions, especially in this century. But, fortunately, there are some ways to help you maintain your focus.

1. *Define the task.* The first step is to identify what job you want to focus on. For example, you may need to build a ten-page PowerPoint deck for an upcoming meeting. Or, you may want to learn a new skill before a month. It is understanding what to do that gives you a clear sense of direction. It reduces ambiguity and increases focus.

2. *Create a working environment.* Gaining attention in a cluttered and noisy room can prove challenging. That's why it is essential to have a study room that allows for a total focus. Keep your desk clean and tidy, and remove anything that might distract you. If your task is to read a book for one hour after you come back from school or work, make sure to put the writing on the desk, and anything you might need—a marker, a bottle of water to prepare you for the reading without any interruptions. If you are going to be practising for a speech, you should have an environment that is as close as possible to the actual situation you will be in when delivering the speech. The key is to achieve more by having the tool and workspace you need ready to maximize your time and effort.

3. *Remove all distractions.* When working on a particular task, it's essential to remove all distractions caused by technology (i.e., social network app, instant messaging, pop-up notifications, television, or computer). Make sure to turn off all visual and audible information. Close all applications except the one that is important for the task. Turn off your phone, or at least mute it.

4. *Have a focus session.* Some jobs are simply too big or complex to complete in a single session, and most people have a limit as to how long they can focus on a single task before they hit mental exhaustion. I suggest that most people start with a twenty-five minutes focus session, followed by a five minutes break. It may not sound like a lot, but you will be surprised at how challenging staying fully focused for twenty-five minutes can be. As you improve your focus, you will find that you can increase your focus session, perhaps to thirty, forty, or even fifty minutes.

5. *Choose your moments.* Are you a night owl or a morning lark? Night owls are people that majorly sleep late (around 2 a.m.) and wake up late (around 10 a.m.). On the other hand, morning larks are people that sleep

early (around 10 p.m.) and wake up early (around 6 a.m.). Not everyone functions or works the same way. Some people tend to be more energetic and active during the early morning, which decreases throughout the day, while some are more productive and focused during mid-day. Also, depending on the type of work you do, your circumstances might be different. Be aware of what time of the day your mind becomes more active and take advantage of that to work on a task that demands your attention. Leave repetitive work for the lower-energy moment.

6. *Reward yourself*: Reward yourself whenever you complete a task. Do things that relieve you or make you happy such as watching your favourite show, buying yourself something, spending time with a close friend, or cooking your favourite food.

Benefits of being focused

There are a lot of benefits to being focused, but here are a few.

1. *It reduces stress.* When we are overwhelmed with tasks and are unable to prioritize the job that's important to us and focus on it, our stress level will increase drastically. As you develop clarity and understand what is crucial for you, this allows you to get things done and positively impact your stress level. When you focus on what is not essential, all your efforts lead to nothing, which can increase your frustration, thereby, increasing your stress.

2. *It increases momentum.* When you focus on a single task, you increase your effectiveness without distraction, which helps you make more and faster progress. When you can focus on a single task, such as writing a blog post, and you can complete it before the appointed deadline, it increases morale. Getting things done at the right time is what everybody wants, including your boss. As your team starts to see progress being made, it motivates them to work harder, as they can see the results of their effort, which helps the team build momentum.

3. *Allow for better quality work.* Getting yourself to do an excellent job

on a task isn't about increasing the time you spend on a project but about providing quality work in a shorter time. By giving all your attention to a task, you are more likely to get the job done quicker and even better. Focusing on a task allows your brain to work and develop new ideas associated with the task. Even during break, your mind will subconsciously be working on the job. It is excellent for artists, designers, researchers, executives, and writers, and those who want to innovate.

Focus is a vital ingredient to the success of our life. When distracted, always realize and bring yourself back to what's essential. Remember: Whatever you focus on will multiply, be it good or bad.

Habit

Who we are right now and what we do is all based on the practices we've made for ourselves. Our habits control our lives. Many folks are what they are right now because of their daily decisions and attitude, and behaviours that have become a habit.

Habit is the repetitive and persistent action you take. During our adolescence, we've learned to do various activities automatically. Adolescents learned to brush their teeth day and night, dress after bathing, and play with friends all day without rational thinking. If you love to always chew crunchy snacks when watching a movie, or finger biting when stressed or enjoy working out each morning, that is because you've made it a habit. You've conditioned your mind and body to do these activities with little conscious energy.

Habits are "autopilot" behaviours that can save your mental energy for creative problem-solving. To become successful, you need good habits. Many people are not who they want to be, and continue to live a life of dissatisfaction by the pressure of their work. The problem is that they fail to establish the necessary habits needed to live a successful and productive life. All successful people have consistent daily habits that make them productive and achieve more. When you focus on a particular activity or character, and you put in constant effort, it later becomes a habit.

Habit shapes your life far more than you probably realize. About forty-five percent of the actions you perform each day aren't actual decisions, but habits. Some of us have created the habits of drinking coffee just after waking, habits of spending lavishly, habits of drinking too much alcohol, habits of reading each day, habits of praying before going to bed, habits of eating healthy. The more you do things consistently, the more it becomes automatic.

A habit is a crucial tool for growth. Think about it: the reason you were able to ride a bike or drive a car comfortably is because of the consistent, daily effort and practice. Over time, your daily practice later became a habit that makes it less energy-consuming and natural to drive a car or ride a bike. Having a habit that makes you productive is good, but when you develop a terrible habit, it can be challenging to change.

The Psychology of Habit

The habit starts with a psychological pattern that Charles Duhigg, a reporter for the New York Times and author of *The Power of Habit*, refers to as a "habit loop." The habit loop is a three-part process: cue, routine, and reward.

The cue or trigger tells the brain to go into automatic mode and let a behaviour unfold. The routine is the behaviour itself. It is what we do that morphs into habits. The reward is the satisfied feeling we get when we've completed a routine that allows the brain to remember the "habit loop" in the future. Neuroscientists have traced our habit-making behaviours to a part of the brain called the basal ganglia, which play a crucial role in the development of emotions, memories, and pattern recognition.

Meanwhile, a decision is made in a different part of the brain called the prefrontal cortex. When a behaviour becomes automatic, it no longer controls the conscious thought, but the subconscious thinking, which allows the decision-making part of the brain to get into a kind of sleep-mode. "In fact, the brain starts working less and less," says Duhigg. "The brain can almost completely shut down...And this is a real advantage because it means you have all of this mental activity you can devote to something else." Haven't you had the experience of driving or walking, but not being aware of it until you got to your destination? That's the effect of a habit—it becomes easier, while driving, to focus on something else: the radio, or a conversation you are having. The driving becomes automatic so that you don't need to think about it too much to drive safely. "You can do these complex behaviours without being mentally aware of it all," Duhigg says. "And that's because of the capacity of our basal ganglia: to take a behaviour and turn it into an automatic routine."

Studies have shown that people will perform automated behaviours, like brushing their teeth, the same way, every single time they're in the same environment. But when they change location, the behaviour likely changes. Once the cue or trigger changes, the habit begins to break. Duhigg said, "If you want to quit smoking, you should stop smoking while you're on vacation because all your old cues and old rewards aren't there anymore. So you have this ability to form a new pattern and hopefully be able to carry it over into your life."

Everyone has habits—some are positive, and others are not. To be successful and achieve more, you have to develop a habit loop that would contribute to your success. Developing good habits is difficult as they are usually not fun, but it is worth it. Your habit changes and determines your identity. If you want to be a writer, singer, fighter, salesperson, or mentor, you have to develop habits associated with those professions. By creating good habits and adopting positive behaviours, you too can become successful. Aristotle said: "We are what we repeatedly do. Excellence, then, is not an act but a habit." Here are some of the habits that most successful people have in common that you can adopt in your life.

1. *They get up early.* Waking up early is one of the best ways to get things done. When you build the habit of waking up early than everyone else, you have more time to spend and less noise to work on essential tasks. About fifty percent of the self-made millionaires in Corley's research got out of bed at least three hours before their workday started. "Getting

up at five in the morning to tackle the top three things you want to accomplish in your day allows you to regain control of your life," he wrote. "It gives you a sense of confidence that you, indeed, direct your life." Those who wake up early tend to have more free time to spend with family and personal projects.

2. *They read a lot.* Reading is undoubtedly an excellent habit to cultivate in your life. According to research from Thomas Crowley, eighty-five percent of self-made millionaires read two or more books per month. Most of them read self-help books, biographies, and history. Reading biographies of people is fundamental to help you learn life lessons of perhaps more experienced people. The investor mastermind, Warren Buffett, says that reading has been the most crucial habit he has developed.

3. *They spend fifteen to thirty minutes each day on focused thinking.* Many successful people spend some of their time each day meditating on their personal and professional life. Often they'll reflect on their career, their health, and relationships. Having quiet time to analyze your thoughts is associated with stress reduction. You can use this minute to relax your body as it can help recover your strength and relax your brain.

4. *They are goal-oriented.* You need to have a goal to achieve success. You need to set goals and put in your consistent effort to work on them, forming daily habits. All highly successful people are goal-oriented. They are obsessed with pursuing their goals and often refer to both short- and long-term goals. "They know exactly what they want," Brain Tracy wrote, "they have it written down, they have written plans to accomplish it, and they both review and work on their plans as a daily routine."

To further elaborate:

Cue or trigger: A location, certain people, a particular object, or an emotional state.

Routine: Watching TV, smoking a cigarette, eating snacks, biting your nails.

Reward: The pleasure chemical released in the brain reinforces the habit loop.

Habits reduce cognitive loads, free up capacity, and allow you to focus on essential tasks or process any new information that comes in.

Goal Setting

Setting goals is an essential ingredient to success and everyone has goals to achieve; for example, yours might be to write a book, lose weight, or become the boss of your own. These goals can also be set for various intervals: daily, weekly, monthly, or yearly. Goal setting gives you the precision to aim/target, which increases focus, hence, result in greater accomplishments. It brings clarity to your ambitions. There is nothing worse than working on a project without knowing its purpose or what it is contributing. With a goal in sight, projects take on more meaning and purpose. I remember when I gave myself the goal to write the book you're currently reading, I gave myself a reasonable starting and an ending date. When the date was clearly defined, I never missed a day without writing. The moment my goal was clearly stated, it brought me more focus and determination which led to the completion of the book.

To become productive in your personal and professional life, you need to have goals. Breaking down broad goals into small achievable, individual goals makes it easier for you to achieve results across a given time frame. Setting a timeframe to complete this book was the "magic" I needed to complete this book and other tasks. Having goals in your business guides your employees to do what's essential, which increases the company's productivity. The importance of goal setting can't be overstated.

Research has found that setting healthy goals boosts performance by motivating people to increase their effort, inducing sharper focus, and prioritizing. A study found that setting meaningful goals in the business allows people to work faster at completing their tasks irrespective of financial rewards. Your goals keep you moving forward and prepare you for success. Goals give your life a sense of purpose.

Here are some things goals can help you with within your business or hobby.

1. *Goals trigger behaviour.* Having clear, compelling goals mobilizes your focus towards actionable practices. It pushes you to take the initiative of getting things done. Let's assume, for example, Clifford has the goal of creating a blog. You ask him what his blog would be about, and he responds, "Anything." Do you think that would be enough to motivate Clifford? I doubt that. The issue is Clifford isn't precise enough about his blog. Conversely, supposing Clifford was able to state what his blog would be about (i.e., photography, cooking, tech, or fashion trends) and how much it will cost to make it running. The moment he can figure this out, he becomes focused, which triggers him to act.

2. *Goals guide your attention.* There would be nothing to focus on if there's never a goal. Setting goals activates your conscious mind to focus on the task at hand. When you become aware and focused on a mission, your mind and body invest their energy to accomplish it. There's a Tony Robbins saying, "Where focus goes, energy flows." Goals remove confusion and guesses. Both young and old folks with an ingrained goal keep themselves on course to reach their point of aim. Let your goals direct your focus.

3. *Goals sustain momentum.* Achieving goals is a thrilling experience as they lead to the results you want. Successful people who set and achieve goals don't ever want to stop setting goals because of the progress they get. It motivates you to do more as the brain releases dopamine—a happy hormone—when it gets what it wants. It allows you to push yourself more and set higher goals as the brain gets rewarded. That's why most high achievers don't stop working hard and setting audacious goals for themselves.

4. *Goals help to establish limits.* People with goals can prioritize what is important to them and abstain from what is not. They associate more with people who would help achieve their goals and are not influenced by people who would stop them. Goal setting allows you to set boundaries in life. You can define your limits and help you eliminate distractions. What should matter to you are the goals you set, and therefore, anything that doesn't contribute to it should be considered a distraction.

How Goal Setting Improves your Brain

Goal setting doesn't just make you achieve more, but it also changes your brain's structure. A study in Behavioral and Cognition Neuroscience Reviews showed that when you set goals, multiple parts of the brain become engaged:

1. The amygdala, which is the brain's emotional centre, evaluates how important the goal is to you.
2. The frontal lobe, responsible for solving problems in the brain, defines the specifics of the goal.
3. Amygdala and the frontal lobe then work together to keep you focused on the completion of your goal.

Because of the brain's neuroplasticity—the ability to undergo structural and physiological change—it changes its structure to help you optimize behaviours and tasks. This phenomenon was first identified in a study of multiple sclerosis patients at the University of Texas. Multiple Sclerosis (MS) is a severe degenerative disease of the brain with symptoms like numbness, loss of muscular coordination, speech impairment, and severe fatigue.

The study showed that MS patients' symptoms were lessened when goals were set and achieved. In effect, goal setting healed their brain. A study published in the Journal of Experiment Psychology showed that people who formed an ambitious goal often make it. People who created an easier goal failed to achieve it. Ambitious goals are far more motivating as they stimulate the brain more than easily achieved goals. The Psychological Bulletin said ninety percent of the studies showed that more challenging goals led to higher performance. More manageable goals or "do your best" goals did not affect the brain or the person's ability to achieve their goals. The article reported, "Goal setting is most likely to improve task performance when the goals are specific and sufficiently challenging."

It should be noted that the brain's ability to change its structure occurs only when the individual is setting the goal. The neuroplasticity of the brain won't happen when your boss or other people set the goal for you. Inc. reports, "All a leader can do is having ambitious, challenging goals for themselves in the hope it will inspire others to do the same."

Importance of Goal Setting in Children and Students

Teaching students how to set goals is an essential skill as it proves useful for them in the future. Experts believe that it's the role of educators to help students set short- and long-term goals, which is great to allow students or learners to achieve success outside of the school environment. According to Isaac Ddumba, a teacher at La Colombiere School, encouraging students to set academic and non-academic goals is what's missing in the system. Students and learners who are taught the importance of goals and goal setting tend to achieve more in the future than their peers who did not set goals. The process should start as early as childhood to enable them to set their targets and work towards achieving the goals.

Ddumba notes that goals may range from home or school activities to community actions, among others. He explains that in due course, goal setting can help develop numerous abilities, such as leadership skills, team building, teamwork, accountability, and overcoming challenges, which are all vital in and out of school. Teachers can also play an essential role in helping students foster the habit of setting goals in and out of school. For instance, when a student can complete a specific goal given to him or her, the teacher rewards them with the following:

- Use the teacher's chair
- Take home a class game for a night
- Take a homework pass
- Sit with a friend
- Pick a game at recess
- Choose any class job for the week
- Draw on the chalkboard
- Do half of an assignment
- Teach the class a favourite game
- Have lunch with the principal

- Good behaviour letter sent home

When students develop the habits of setting goals, they become aware of deadlines and increase their focus, which will be applied in their area of work after school.

As the job market becomes competitive, it is vital to encourage students to achieve their goals. Students who set goals for themselves are more accountable for every action or step they take. They are also motivated to try out different fields of study; from this, even students that didn't know their talents can pick an interest.

Julius Zigama, an entrepreneur, said: "Having goals makes learners aware of their actions, efforts, and even time management skills. Setting goals obligates them to take action, regardless of the obstacles that may be in place. As such, it encourages students to develop critical thinking skills, new problem-solving techniques, and a better understanding of how to overcome issues." Goal setting encourages students to track their previous accomplishments and failures and the areas that need improvement. Students who adopt the habit of goal setting focus more on what's essential to their life and achieve long-term success, which motivates them to push forward even when they feel like giving up.

Parents should expose their children to as many opportunities as possible to give them a chance to develop an interest in new areas. Schools should organize events and occasions where successful people are invited as motivational or inspirational speakers. These successful people could be the driving force and proof the students need to believe in themselves and set a goal to achieve their level of success. Goals are fundamental. They are the driving force of growth and productivity.

When you set goals, make sure to: First, be specific about what you want. Let's assume, for instance, you want more money, don't just write "I want more money," instead write precisely how much money you need. If it's a fitness goal, don't just write, "I want a better body," instead write the exact weight or body mass index (BMI) you must reach. Second, be clear about when you must have it. For example, "I will make $1 million every year by

31st December 2020." "I will lose thirty percent of body fat by 30th October 2020." Third, define how you will reach that goal. For example, "I will make $1 million every year by 31st December 2020, doing X, and to do that, I will first need to learn Y and complete Z."

By being clear about WHAT you want, WHEN you must have it, and HOW to achieve the goal, sets your brain to focus on what you need to do to reach that goal. Ensure the goals are meaningful and essential to you as they will get you excited and motivated to achieve your targets.

Act

"You don't have to be great to start, but you do have to start to be great." – Zig Ziglar.

About two years ago, while I was still in college, I was preparing for a math exam—which admittedly, I wasn't good at. But weeks before the exam, during a break, my collegemate would, sort of, gather themselves to the library or somewhere quiet to study math for the preparation of the exam. They would invite me to the group, but often, because of my phobia for math and anything arithmetic, I would decline or only spend a fraction of the time they would normally spend.

So, the exam drew closer and closer until ... Bam!—it was two days before the exam. Realizing this, my mind and heart raced like a cheetah on steroids because I knew if I blew this up my parents would kill me (figuratively!). Because of that, I choose to forcibly bring out every inner motivation and focus I got so I don't fail. On a typical day, I normally give up about thirty minutes of my time studying for whatever test or exam I have, but this time was different—I literally spent four hours dedicated to studying.

In a nutshell, after taking the exam, I scored a total of 66/100. That was a phenomenal score for me. However, at that moment it hit me, supposedly I had practised for the math exam a week or two prior to the exam, I could have gotten a score that's over 70, 75, or even 80. But another interesting thing I observed was, if I hadn't read two days before the exam, I would have received a lower score that would have ruined me. That moment, I learned a pretty good lesson—no matter what, always choose to act.

Too often, a large chunk of people spends the majority of their time thinking, procrastinating, researching every aspect and debating about the pros and cons rather than just doing it. The attitude of not acting is very prevalent in our relationship, social, and business life. Let's say, for instance, you are in a board meeting and a great idea lit up in your mind, rather than speaking up, you stop instead. The "overthinking mindset" is not only dangerous (as it can make you lose opportunities), but, also, it is largely harmful to a company itself. You need to develop the "action mindset."

Companies are occupied with "experts" who spend more time thinking, looking at the data and stats, debating with other "experts" if the former approach is better than the latter. This does not only stall the company's growth but eventually makes the company non-existent.

Debating on what's right or wrong, good or bad, doesn't bring profit. Action does. The economist and author of The Complacent Class, Tyler Cowen, emphasizes more on the attitude of over-thinking, "The more information that is out there, the greater the returns to just being willing to sit down and apply yourself. Information isn't what's scarce; it is the willingness to do something with it." This brings me to a very popular quote we all know, "Knowledge is power." Well, that is not true. Let's look at it from this point of view, if knowledge was truly power that would mean anybody with a device to access the vast sea of knowledge on the internet would be successful, easily.

Yet, that's not the case.

The only powerful thing that truly brings success is action. We all have goals and dreams to achieve. Some are more than the other. However, one of the easiest ways people tend to kill their dream is by overthinking it. You spend way too much time doing the planning and preparation, trying to make it perfect, day-dreaming what the result is going to be if you begin to work on it or how much you could earn if you could just get a store or distributor...and this "wandering thoughts" keeps on going until you either lose motivation, or someone beats you to it.

The problem is we are always waiting for things to be perfect, we are always getting advice from different people with diverse opinions; but guess what, things are never going to be perfect, and the advice you receive from people will not give you clarity on what to do, rather, it confuses you on what to do. The solution to the "overthinking mindset" is to stop thinking and just do it. Dr. Martin Luther King Jr. once said, "Take the first step in faith. You don't have to see the whole staircase, just take the first step." Peter Marshall, a television personality, also said, "Small deeds done are better than great deeds planned."

The key here is not to think about it but do it. When you find yourself overthinking, or debating on the pros and cons of it, take a step back from those thoughts and focus on the one important thing, and just do it.

Overthinking with your health

Do you think the act of overthinking doesn't affect your health? If yes, you're wrong. According to Susan Nolen-Hoeksenma's ground-breaking research, she noticed that overthinking affects our physical and emotional health. Overthinking leads to depression. And she also found that most women do too much thinking. Here are some of her findings:

- Those who over-think are more susceptible to severe depression and anxiety— especially in women—and interfere with good problem-solving.
- Overthinking is a national epidemic among young and middle-aged adults but is relatively rare among older adults: 73% of 25-35 years-olds over-thinks compared to 52% of 45-55 years-olds and just 20% of 65-75 years-olds.
- Women are significantly more likely than men to fall into overthinking and to be immobilized by it: 57% of women and 43% of men are over-thinkers.
- Overthinkers are significantly more likely to abuse drugs and alcohol, and overthinking may push some individuals to consider or attempt suicide.

You might be familiar with the word, "How we think determines how we live."

Because of the power our mind possesses, it's only wise to use it responsibly. A few years back, while I was watching an interview with Steve Jobs, I got to notice why he chose to always wear a black turtleneck, blue jeans, and balance sneakers—every day. The reason was he didn't want to spend most of his time and "brain juice" thinking about what outfit to wear each morning.

Not long later, I read an article about how Elizabeth Holmes, the founder of the infamous blood-testing startup called Theranos, also wears only a black turtleneck and suit just for the same reason as Jobs. Both Jobs and Holmes were trying to limit their thinking on the trivial stuff of their life to focus more on what's important. I'm not suggesting you too should have a single dress code that you wear every day. I believe there are better ways to think less and do more.

1. Stay in the present. Many people fail to take action now all because of the terrible experience they had in the past. Studies have shown that adults who have a phobia for public speaking, or phobia for asking questions, or a phobia of giving opinion behave that way because of the childhood rejection they had at school or home. Teachers or parents who don't embrace the practice of children asking questions or trying new things will only breed future adults that become discouraged to act. The majority of people who failed their first business usually default to being an employee just because they let their experience of failing to hold them down from creating a new and better venture. A wise man said, "The past is not a place to live, but a place to learn." The moment you understand that and begin to focus on the positive side of the future, that is when you can be able to act with greater confidence.

2. Don't pollute your mind with too much information. Why is too much information a bad thing? Isn't that what all of us should be striving for (so that robots won't take our jobs?) Let me share with you a personal experience. Before I had any functional savings or knew anything about money, I took it upon myself to learn some of the ways I could earn money. I didn't want to be left behind. Like anyone would do, I went to Google and typed in the keywords, "How do I make money." Not

surprised, I got a ton of information concerning ways I could earn money, including passive and active incomes. I found information on real estate, stock investing, FOREX trading, web design, app development, affiliate marketing, and so many more. At first, I was thrilled to find out that there are many ways I could make money, but as days went by, I couldn't find a sure-fire way of making money. I later became overwhelmed and couldn't decide which to focus on. This process continued for over a year—I kept on living my life with lots of information but with no action. So a friend of mine who was doing well in real estate advised me to put my brainpower into a single niche. Then and there, I thought within myself what I was good at and love doing, which was writing and marketing, so I spent a lot of my time learning the craft of writing. After that, I worked my way up to marketing. The result of those actions has been terrific. If I had continued to populate my brain with excess information, I would have probably been brain dead. The point is: focus on one thing that's most important for you to accomplish that day, month, or year, and then work your way up.

3. Don't wait until conditions are perfect, because they won't. The vast majority of the world's population is seeking perfection. The main reason people choose to do butt augmentation, breast implant, jaw restructuring, Botox, and other cosmetic procedures is that they seek absolute perfection. But the reality is, nothing is ever perfect (especially that made from humans). Many businesses fail to progress all for the reason that they are waiting for the "perfect" market condition, or to have the "perfect" facilities, or the "perfect" employees, which, to many businesses surprise, will never occur. If you are always seeking the "perfect" conditions to get started, you will be waiting till eternity. You must take action now and make the proper adjustments and changes as you move ahead. No one can ever fully be prepared for what the future holds—it is unknown. The only thing you should be worried about is what happens now and how you handle it. As Salvador Dali perfectly puts it, "Have no fear of perfection—you'll never reach it."

4. Just take action! Tony Robbins said, "The only impossible journey is

the one you never begin." The only thing stopping you from doing that which you want to do is the fear you have allowed to dominate your mind and body. The cure to that fear is: Action! If you are running a business, rather than dwelling in that fear, just take action. If you find yourself close to an exam or test, rather than convincing yourself of how lacklustre your performance has been, just start reading. If you find yourself in front of people to make a public presentation, rather than thinking how awful you'll sound, just speak and don't stop speaking (except if necessary). And to end this list, allow me to borrow a quote from Mario Cuomo who said, "There are only two rules for being successful. One, figure out exactly what you want to do, and two, do it." My quote to you: Just take action!

Take the Leap and Embrace It

Every second you spend overplanning, you lose the opportunity to get a result. Notice that I used the word "overplanning". There's nothing wrong with planning or trying to get enough data and information about a particular task before venturing into it. However, the real issue comes, like every other thing, when it becomes chronic. Allow me to cite an analogy. Many of us view stress with a negative connotation, but stress is a good thing.

Stress is an evolutionary tool that has been passed down from our prehistoric ancestors for our safety. When threatened or faced with a predator, our ancestors used to stress to either fight or flee from a perilous situation. Stress increases our blood pressure, increases our glucose level to provide the energy necessary to flee or fight, and it also increases our focus to be aware of threats. This trait has proven useful for our survival, which is the primary reason it has been passed down through the gene from generation to generation. However, stress becomes perilous when it becomes incessant. For example, consuming sugar is necessary for our body to function as sugar serves as a form of energy, however, when it becomes "too much", it can be harmful to your health.

In the wild, our ancestors only needed the effect of stress for a short period after the threat was over. But in the 21st-century world, various things continuously causes us stress—job interviews, exams, public speaking, 9-to-5 job, and even taking care of children. All of these stress-inducing activities constantly raise our stress level till it becomes chronic and very harmful to our well-being.

Planning is also a good thing as it involves doing proper research that reduces risk and the chance of failing. However, when planning becomes chronic—overplanning—that's when it becomes bad. The time you spend on overplanning should be spent on taking action. Don't over-plan and under-act. It doesn't matter what you want to venture into or how difficult it might seem, there's one thing that's common to all successful brands and people: They take the first step.

One of the most commonly used phrases is, "I want to ________." For example, "I want to lose 30 pounds," "I want to earn more money," "I want to own a house," and so on. But many of those phrases are never actually fulfilled. People just talk, ponder, and debate, but do little to nothing to make it happen. You have to understand that words don't make results. Every product or technology that has ever existed all started as an idea, but it took action to make it into a reality. Every war that ever existed began with a gruesome idea to kill; every peace that ever began also started as an idea to bring resolution to the world, but the action made it a reality. You are what you do, not what you say.

One of the most intriguing things that I've noticed about inaction is that it's more exhausting and debilitating than action. Whenever I break through the fear of speaking in public, speaking my opinion in a class, or anything, it feels exhilarating, which only allows me to do more of it. But when I fail to take action on speaking out my opinion, or anything, throughout that day I won't feel comfortable because I know I had something important to say, but I allowed my fear to take control of me. You have felt that way also, right? Good, because everyone has.

Even though we humans tend to avoid situations that involve us taking responsibility and control of the outcome, we feel way worse when we don't do it (especially when we know it's important). So, to ease yourself from that baggage of self-guilt (feelings of pain and regret), it is best for you to take the easier and exhilarating road of action. Action is the creator of results.

Rest

I hope before now you've always prioritized rest. Rest is essential not only for your health, happiness, and relationships but also for your productivity. To be productive, it's not just enough to have a personal organizing system, functioning correctly. Adequate rest is a critical practice to cultivate that can help you regain focus and energy to handle every task at hand. Without proper relaxation, a job that, on a typical day, you could finish within an hour will be stretched to three hours. Like I have always said, we live in a world that is becoming busier than ever, a large proportion of people are overwhelmed and stressed out by the intense pressure (sometimes, from ourselves) and workload of modern life. There are numerous distractions and demands for our attention and energy. When we are stressed or tired, we often neglect the option of taking a break even when we cannot think clearly or progress with our work anymore. The smart thing to do at this point is to rest.

Resting is essential if you want to be more productive, competent, and happier. And it's not only about sleeping well at night. Studies have proven that taking short breaks very often throughout the day is very beneficial to our performance and growth. The human body isn't designed to work like a machine. It needs time for recovery to regain its strength to become more productive. After each break, we renew our body's energy, reactivate our brain, and handle any task with more focus and motivation. Many schools and businesses haven't understood the importance of proper resting in students' and employees' performance and health. When the mind gets overworked without recovery, it affects the body as a whole. A tired brain makes you susceptible to sickness that can cause you to miss days from work or school. A relaxed mind and body, even for an hour, restore your depleted energy, improves focus, repairs your body, increases your creativity, and improves mood. To get the most out of your break or rest session, you can do some of these practices.

1. *Take an ice bath.* Ice baths can do wonders for your body and have you feeling rejuvenated physically. There's a reason why so many professional athletes use ice baths as a way to recover. If you find yourself feeling worn down, this technique may do just the trick, especially if you're proactive about the treatment.

2. *Take a warm bath.* If the ice bath sounds too much for you to bear, warm baths can help you relax in different ways. Warm baths can help ease anxiety, soothe your skin, and even make it easier to fall asleep—if that's what you want.

3. *Take breaks on a micro and macro level.* Everyone needs time to recoup and recharge. It can be as easy as sitting outside for a few minutes before going back to work, taking one day to yourself a week, or a relaxing vacation. If you keep pushing yourself until you start to feel awful or "shut down," it will be harder to recover and rest.

4. *Practice not thinking.* We are creatures who can't do without thinking. We think about a lot of things (i.e., what to wear, what to say, what to do next). But too much thinking is exhausting and bad for our health when done repeatedly without proper breaks to help us recover our minds from bothering thoughts. Open your senses to what is happening around you and pay attention, but don't think about them. Just experience them.

5. *Listen to instrumental music or ambient noise.* Sounds like running water, birds chirping, and even storms can help you relax and stop stressing about whatever is going on through your head. You can find playlists of these kinds on the internet.

6. *Stay away from electronics, particularly at night when trying to rest.* Your electronic device's screen emits blue lights that affect your sleep-wake cycle. If you're having trouble feeling well-rested, electronics might be a part of the problem.

Because of the popularity of "smartphone" breaks, research was done that focused on whether taking a break with a smartphone (e.g., browsing the internet or using social network services) has a different association with regaining strength after a regular break, i.e., walking, or chatting face-to-face with friends. The result showed that psychological detachments by breaks, independent of break modes, did increase vigor and reduce emotional exhaustion. However, the study also found that the effects, particularly in lowering emotional fatigue, were significantly lower for smartphone break groups versus the conventional group.

Relaxing and involving yourself in activities of your preference that probably have nothing to do with your job, helps you become better at work. Spending a day or two each week on events not related to work allows you to create new ideas and reduce stress. The thoughts of many people are that resting is for people who aren't determined to achieve greatness. But that's not true. Contrary to that, ambitious people tend to rest more by connecting more with nature and the outdoors, allowing the beauty of the environment and the opportunities that life offers, such as hiking, surfing, skiing, and climbing, to replenish their energy.

You must establish short cycle breaks that adapt to your body. And you have to understand your body, to decide what length of break would be most effective for you. You must understand your strength and adjust your activities to it, not the other way round. Know this: If you get tired, learn to rest, not quit.

8

Principle #8: The Five Rules Of Successful Living

Either you deal with what is the reality, or you can be sure that the reality is going to deal with you. — Alex Haley.

Life can be tricky for a lot of people. Everyone's experience of life is different. For some people, life is tough; for others, life is easy and pleasurable. Some people were able to succeed at an early age; for others, it took them ages to accomplish success. Some people were able to get things right with just a single try; for others, it took them lots of trying. Some were able to discover their purpose earlier in life, while others, much later. To achieve remarkable accomplishments and success, you have to understand specific rules that will guide you to deal with life better and achieve more. These rules are consistent with the way most high achievers handle situations and live fulfilling lives.

Rule One
Take Responsibility

Being responsible is an essential character of great leaders, and it is a critical factor for their success. For many folks, everything wrong that happens to them is always someone else's fault. But that's not the right way to live a good life. You must be able to take full responsibility for your life. Taking responsibility gives you a remarkable professional life, but it also builds trust with the people you associate with. It is easier not to be responsible for your actions and make excuses because those we work with are so closely intertwined and dependent on others in our activities. When you ask people the reasons for their failure or shortcomings, many will tend to shift the blame away from themselves to someone else. Words like, "It's the government's fault," "My boss wasn't nice to me," "My parents didn't provide me with the right education," "The teacher wasn't good enough," have become common excuses most people make when trying to blame others.

Taking personal responsibility for whatever happens to you is a crucial step in becoming more than yourself. It takes courage, acceptance, and a realistic view of your life circumstances to become responsible. People who take full responsibility for their life experience more control, happiness, and are trustworthy. They can make choices because they understand that they are responsible for their decisions. Let's illustrate this with a story.

Jane, a 25-year-old, works in a coffee shop to earn money and sustain herself since she no longer stays with her parents. When Jane was in college, in her 3rd year, she was compelled to drop out because her parents couldn't finance her college. Jane's parents aren't the wealthy type but worked tirelessly to feed and send their children to school. Jane was devastated by what was happening to her. She thought that her dream of becoming a prolific writer was reduced to ruins. She went to her parents and blamed them for her downfall and how things could have been better if she could continue her education.

Her parents were crushed. They were sad and disappointed by her remarks because they had worked so hard to cater for Jane and her siblings to school. She later decided to go for a job interview and then got a job at a coffee shop.

Five years later, she noticed a long-time college mate walk into the shop. We will call Jane's college mate, Noah. Noah was neatly dressed and had a nice, black mustang. Although Jane wasn't pleased with her job, she was, nevertheless, surprised and ecstatic to meet him. Later that day, she and Noah spent a few hours together, discussing. Jane explained her story to

Noah: how her parents were the cause of her current situation.

Noah said something that widened her eyes. He told her that a year after she dropped out, he also did the same. Her eyebrows were raised; her mouth slightly opened. She stuttered as she asked, "What happened?" "How did you get so successful, then?"

Noah smiled.

"I worked on myself and took responsibility for my life," he responded. "I dropped out of college and spent most of my time learning and growing my craft—social media marketing. That led me to create success. I didn't make excuses or blamed anyone for what happened to me." Jane couldn't believe her ears. She had been blaming others for her misfortune. Since that sudden enlightenment, Jane began spending more time studying, attending seminars, and attending online classes to help her become a better writer. Close to three years later, she completed the first book that got her a book contract of $50,000.

She was astounded by the experience. She regretted wasting many years blaming others and doing nothing about her dream. She apologized to her parents for her ignorance and lackadaisical attitude.

Just about everyone agrees that taking responsibility is an essential trait of success. Likewise, Jane was only able to get her life back on track when she realized that the events happening in her life were the result of her choices. It's neither your parents' fault, nor the government's fault that you couldn't succeed, but your fault for not taking massive responsibility for your actions and decisions. Though the government might have caused a hindrance to your progress, ultimately, it's up to you to make the right choices that result in success.

To take accountability for your life is to acknowledge that your life is your responsibility and yours alone. You are in charge of your life. If you want to be a writer, then be a writer. Your parents, spouse, friend, the climate isn't the cause of your predicament. It's you. It's always you versus you. Want to be a lawyer? Then be a lawyer. Want to be a good spouse? Then be a good spouse. Want to be fit? Then eat healthy and exercise regularly. When you want something in your life or become a certain kind of person, put in the work required to achieve that; and take full ownership of every action and circumstance in your life. You alone can decide what you want.

Failure to accept personal responsibility may be of benefit to you on occasion or in the short-term. Making excuses for your misdeed may save you at that time, but eventually, this poor choice will catch up with you, and it will typically lead to more pain down the road.

A person who admits his or her wrongdoings, or acknowledges the decisions made has a leader's character. All great leaders don't complain or blame others for their circumstances but immediately recognize the reality and find ways to fix it. Learning to take on responsibility in your personal and business life can be difficult. But it's a valuable activity to do that which can significantly transform your life. Don't make excuses. People who do, rather than being accountable for their thoughts, actions, and goals will fail to succeed in their lives compared to those who don't make excuses and complain.

People don't desire to take responsibilities or leadership roles for specific reasons ranging from: fear of failure, laziness, not being confident, not feeling they have the authority, or not seeing others (especially leaders or people they care about) modelling accountability. Whatever the reason might be, if you fail to be accountable, you'll fail in your business, fail as a team member, fail as a spouse. You will fail to grow as an individual, which makes it more important to be responsible. There are some common signs people display when they become irresponsible. These include:

- Avoiding taking the initiative and being dependent on others for work, advice, and instructions.
- Avoiding challenging tasks and not taking a manageable risk.
- Missing deadlines and meeting.
- Blaming others for mistakes and failures.
- Complain about a lot of things.
- Lacking interest in their work and the well-being of the team.
- Making excuses regularly.

How to Become Responsible

Taking responsibility doesn't just help you believe more; it also enables you to build a stronger relationship with your partner or spouse. Being responsible as with anything isn't innate to us. It is a skill that's learned as we grow and learn through life. Your sense of responsibility can come from your family members, from close-ties, or from something you saw on TV. Since your level of responsibility is dependent on what you see and hear, it means you are susceptible to learn both good and evil characters. But it is still your choice. Whether you choose to be responsible or not, it is you who gets to decide that. No one else. Responsibility is a skill that can be learned and improved based on your own conscious decision. Here are a few behaviors you can adopt to become responsible in your personal and professional life.

1. *Don't make excuses.* Making excuses that the government, friends, or boss are the cause of your misfortune in your relationship or business life isn't going to make you open to others or successful. It only makes you feel like the victim of the circumstances. It's an escape. Excuses might make you feel okay for about a minute, but it won't help you bring your life back together. So before making an excuse, think for a moment, *Will my excuses change the circumstance? Will it make my team or crew build trust with me? Or is it not just an escape to feel safe for a minute?*

2. *Don't complain.* Complaining about how your life sucks, how things are spiralling down, or how you aren't getting anything done isn't going to make you a better life. Taking action will. Want better pay in your job? Bring more value than you use to. Want to lose weight? Go to the gym and eat healthy. Want a better relationship? Then make yourself a better man or woman that the right partner would want to spend his or her life with. Want to stop drinking alcohol? Then stop drinking alcohol. Want to become better in your craft? Then read and study more. It's that simple. Instead of complaining about how things aren't working right, just put in the work and let your actions dictate. Complainers are never happy because of how they think about the things that happen in

their life.

3. *Do things without being told.* You should not be told to clear and tidy your room before you do so. You shouldn't be told to take your bath and brush your teeth twice a day before you do so. Effecting just the things you are asked to do is responsible, but to indicate that you can care for yourself and others around you, you need to do things without being told. That shows you are responsible and competent enough to see what needs to be done and take care of it.

4. *Be consistent with your actions.* Great leaders are not just responsible for a day but consistently. You shouldn't act responsibly on Mondays and Tuesdays, and not responsibly on Thursdays and Fridays. Being responsible is for you to be consistent in your routine and stick to it. For example, when you acquire a task from your boss or promise a friend to come to his event, you should be able to keep to your promise and give one hundred percent of your effort to always handle the task. It proves to people that they can always depend on you.

5. *Manage your finance.* Learning how to save your money and invest it in assets shows that you understand the importance of money and how to manage it. Whatever your situation is in life, whether successful or not, married or single, you should have goals for your money and how to spend it. It would make you confident because you wouldn't need to continually ask friends and relatives for help with cash. Spend your money on your needs—paying your bills, buying groceries, investing in assets—not wants.

Rule Two

Success Takes Time

Things take time. The seeds planted do not sprout the next day, but that doesn't mean they never will. Be patient. Things will unfold for you. — Unknown.

One of our mistakes is thinking that successful people became successful overnight. The Wright brothers didn't invent the world's first motor-operated aeroplane overnight. Steve Harvey didn't begin to earn millions of dollars annually for his show with just a single comedy night. We all want to be the best. We want to have great achievements quickly. Everyone wants to have the best car, have a multi-million dollar house, become fit now, become smart now, or live their dreams right now, but life doesn't work that way.

Good things take time. Great businesses and world-class achievement are not created in a day. It takes time for a child to become an adult. It takes time to become well-groomed. But a lot of us don't realize that for our dreams to be realized; it could take months and years to fully mature. Those who are patient enough to learn all the required skills are those that become great.

Slow and steady progress is the key to extraordinary success. Being patient with your goals and dreams isn't about wasting time doing nothing. On the contrary, it's about taking the time to do things properly. It took about five years to build a space shuttle with lots of rocket design drawings, decades of research, and failed attempts before coming up with the working plans. Depending on the size of a cruise ship, it takes about a year to eighteen months to build one. It can take a year or more to make a movie that we watch in two hours or less.

The point is clear. Everything good in life takes time. It doesn't matter what goal you want to achieve; if it is worth achieving, it will take time. The time it takes is different for each person, depending on certain factors—resources, effort, country, and individual mindset. You may think there is no time to possibly slow down because you have so much that you want to achieve, but look back in your life and acknowledge how much you have already achieved. When we set goals, we want them to be fast and immediate. Nobody wants to waste time or dawdle in their goals; instead, we want everything to happen that instant. This "now" attitude has become a common theme in all parts of life: diet, physical fitness, learning, business, and so on. Let's look at the life of Spencer to understand the power of time.

Spencer lives in Newton, Massachusetts. He has a passion for photography. Spencer always loves to play with the camera that his father bought for him. Spencer was enthusiastic about photography, however, he wasn't able to go to college because he wasn't that good with school activities.

After staying home for some weeks, he decided to visit a very successful photographer who has an office, not far from his place. Spencer located the photographer (let us refer to him as Mr. P) Mr. P invites Spencer to speak with him and explain his situation and interest in photography.

As Spencer got to Mr. P's office, he was welcomed in and asked to sit. Spencer gave a detailed explanation of his life and how things have been bad for him: how his school and social life have gone awry. He explained that his utmost desire is to become a professional photographer as quick as possible.

"How quick do you want to become a professional photographer?" Mr. P asked puzzled.

"A year at most," Spencer responded.

Mr. P giggled as he asked him another question in return.

"How long do you think it took me to achieve great success?"

"A year, I guess," Spencer retorted.

"Eight years. It took me eight years to create a multi-million dollar photography business," says Mr. P.

Spencer's face fell. He couldn't believe it would take that long to really become successful. He didn't know what to say or think.

"To become great," Mr. P says as he looked at Spencer's belittled face, "you have to put in consistent effort for years." Though Spencer was unhappy with how long it could take to become successful, he was willing to put in the work required. "I'm ready to go through the journey and I promise to be diligent and determined and not to waste your time, at all, throughout the training," Spencer says with vigour.

Mr. P was delighted to have Spencer as his mentee and become his coach. He took him under his wings and taught him everything he needed to know to become the best in his craft.

After five years of training, Spencer started his own photography business. He also teaches photography and sells photos on stock photography websites that earn him an annual revenue of about half a million dollars. He realizes that he wouldn't have succeeded if he had rushed things. His years of training led him to great heights. Spencer is now a happy and successful man. He said to me, "Taking my time to learn from Mr. P and not rushing it was the best decision I have ever made. I wouldn't be who I am today without the help of Mr. P and the patience for growth."

Thinking long-term and making steady progress, day-by-day is what produces real results. That is the power of time—when you achieve remarkable success over a long period. With patience, discipline, and hard work, eventually, you'll stumble upon a breakthrough. This approach applies to all areas of our life: art, science, business, design, writing, and so on. If you have a goal that is beyond you, try to slow down rather than speed up. Here are three steps to fully harness the power of slow.

1. *Don't force it.* If you notice your goal is too big and the pace of your growth is slow, so as not to feel frustrated, it's important not to force it. When you set goals, don't expect immediate results because all good things take time to mature. Forcing it only stresses you more, which causes you to quit.

2. *Respect the process.* Mark Zuckerberg became a billionaire at age twenty-three; while, Bill Gates became a billionaire at age thirty-one. Everyone works with a different attitude and mindset that allows some people to achieve success quicker than others. Don't be discouraged if you are not able to learn a craft as quickly as others. Also, don't mock nor demoralize those who aren't able to learn as quickly as you. There's an optimal process that each one of us follows. Respect it.

3. *Make progress.* It doesn't matter how tough or challenging your goals might be, make sure to at least do something daily that pushes you forward. If you want to lose fifty pounds, it is essential not to focus on the full process it takes, instead of the little effort you exhaust daily. What's crucial is progress, not immediacy.

Great goals take time to materialize, and this is a normal process that everyone passes. As long as you put in the work required to move forward, success is inevitable. Take your time. Don't rush it. Engage yourself with the right people. And progress daily.

Rule Three
Failure is Inevitable

I have failed miserably over the past few years. In high school, I failed at becoming the class captain, which I wanted. I also failed to secure a scholarship to college. But I realized that failure was an essential component of my growth. Every time I fail and keep on trying, I always become better. It turned out that my failures were stepping stones for me to reach greater heights. Everyone will fail at some point in their life—including you. Accept it; because it is inevitable.

Whether you are a prodigy or not, gifted or not, talented or not, you will experience failure. Anyone who tells you he/she hasn't failed has never tried anything new. Contrary to many people's ideology, failing can be a positive experience. Think about it: The first time you rode a bicycle, you fell and perhaps got injured. The first time you tried walking like a baby, you fell. The first time you tried stunts or parkour, you fell. But as you kept on falling and falling, your skill improved. Your failures shouldn't discourage you from trying new things, rather it should encourage you. It provides you with knowledge on how to handle a situation better or become more skilled.

The path to success is paved with failure. — Unknown.

High achievers who understand the importance of failure have tapped into its potentials. Many successful companies deliberately seek employees with track records that show both failure and success. People who have failed countless times are usually more experienced in handling certain activities. For example, an engineer who has been working on a project for years with a series of failures, and at the same time, growth, would be better experienced and qualified in doing that work than someone who isn't familiar with the project. Know this: *If you don't fail, you are not even trying.* Making mistakes in your maths test or failing your school project is a learning opportunity for you. Our mistakes and failures allow us to grow. If you don't make mistakes, then there's no need for you to grow. The reason why evolution occurs in the first place is because of the need to evolve. Humans and other animals have been evolving for millions of years and still do because of the need to grow and better adapt to the environment. Successful people use their failures to reinvent themselves.

Successful People that Failed Their Way to Success

Failure is a regular thing. Even the most accomplished of people who control vast empires have failed at some point in their life and still will. But many of these achievers don't let their failure stop them from reaching the dreams. Here are some of the successful people who failed but used their failure as a tool for growth.

Stephen King

King is one of the greatest and prolific writers on Earth. He wrote over sixty novels, many of which are quite long. His writing skills have made him a popular figure. But King wasn't born being a writer. He wrote stories as a teenager and college student, collecting a massive backlog of rejected stories he stored in a large crate. King was working as a teacher in rural Maine when he wrote his first novel, Carrie. By this time, King had some small success selling short stories previously, but nothing that anyone could build a career around. He submitted Carrie thirty times, and he was rejected thirty times. Before his thirty-first attempt, he threw the manuscript out. His wife rescued it from the round file and asked him to try one more time. The rest is history.

George Lucas

Star Wars is one of the highest-grossing movie franchises in Hollywood. Since the release of Episode IV - A New Hope in 1977, the franchise has remained a box office hit. However, Star Wars almost did not make it to the big screen. Three major studios: Disney, United Artists, and Universal all rejected it. Fox backed the movie, hoping that it would be something like American Graffiti, one of the more successful films that Lucas had directed. When shooting Star Wars, nobody got Lucas's vision. There was a lot of tension between him and the actors, the crew, and the executives. Also, Fox had to be creative in its marketing campaign to bring the movie to theatres. However, after its first run, Star Wars instantly became a hit. It changed how movies were made, and the franchise has become a billion-dollar industry.

Albert Einstein

Albert Einstein, arguably the most celebrated theoretical physicist, knows that failures are an essential tool for success. Einstein's genius did not come easy. He had speech difficulties as a child and was once thought to be mentally handicapped. In his teens, he rebelled against his school's reliance on rote learning and failed. He tried to test into Zurich Polytechnic but failed again (although he did well in the math and physics section...as you might expect). Einstein buckled down, received the requisite training, and applied to Zurich Polytechnic again, and was accepted.

A few years later, he had a PhD and was recognized as a leading theorist. A few years after that, he had a Noble Prize for physics and began to be known as the genius of our modern era. He said: *Anyone who has never made a mistake has never tried anything new.*

J.K Rowling

Rowling is the perfect example that success can come to anyone at any time. She is now doing the backstroke through a pool of Harry Potter's money, but that was not always the case. Rowling always planned on being a writer, but life interfered. She battled depression over the untimely death of her mother. Her first marriage failed. She was left trying to provide for herself, raise a young child alone while living on welfare, go to school, and work on a novel in her nonexistent spare time.

Rowling herself said she was the "biggest failure I knew" and credits a lot of her success to her failure. Before Harry Potter became a success, she was a divorced mother, living on welfare, going to school, and writing a novel in her spare time. At a Harvard commencement speech, Rowling had this to say about failure:

"Failure meant stripping away of the inessential. I stopped pretending to myself that I was anything other than what I was, and began to direct all my energy to finish the only work that mattered to me. Had I succeeded at anything else, I might have found the determination to succeed in the one area where I truly belonged. I was set free because my greatest fear had been realized and still alive, and I still had a daughter I adored, and I had an old typewriter and a big idea. And so rock bottom became a solid foundation on which I rebuilt my life."

Michael Jordan

It is hard to imagine it, but Jordan, who is arguably the greatest basketball player ever, was once cut from his high school team. From not being able to stay on his high school team, Jordan kept working and improving. He made the team at North Carolina and became a star college player. Then he played for the Bulls creating an armful of titles.

In the middle of his career, he took a few years off to become a professional baseball player. He ultimately failed in this effort to get to the major leagues but was able to have some good games in the minor league. But even in basketball, where he is the GOAT, he got his success through hard work after failure. As Jordan puts it:

"I have missed more than 9,000 shots in my career. I have lost almost 300 games. On twenty-six occasions I have been entrusted to take the game-winning shot, and I missed. I have failed over and over and over again in my life. And that is why I succeed."

Great achievers owe their success to their mistakes and failures. Without the challenges, rejections, and setbacks they faced, with their persistence and certitude to succeed, they wouldn't have achieved their dreams. To succeed, you have to be willing to fail. Failure is part of the process of success. People who avoid failure also avoid success. Note this: every failed experiment is one step closer to success. Fail often and learn from it. The more you fail, the closer you are to succeed.

There are three things you should know about failure.

1. *Failure hurts.* There's no denying the reality that it is painful when we lose or fail at something. Consistent failure, with a wrong mindset or interpretation, can cause a person to give up trying. It wasn't fun when my online business failed. Failure was heart-wrenching and painful. But

all successful people attribute their success to their darkest moments. It is in this pain that we find the drive to succeed. It might sound like a cliché, but it's true: No pain, no gain.

2. *Failure is inevitable.* You would experience failure just as you experience pain. You can't hide from it. It will come to you. Rather than fighting it, embrace it. Use it as a weapon to succeed. The invention of the electric light-bulb would not have existed without the failures Edison experienced. The mission to the moon would not have been successful without years of errors and challenges. The success of Disney Company was all because of the setbacks Walt Disney faced. Failure is part of the journey to success. Make use of it.

3. *Failure teaches.* People fail for various reasons. Some failed because they didn't put enough effort; some people failed because they had too high expectations; some failed because they did things wrong. Failure provides you with the experience to make better decisions. It pushes you and causes you to grow. It serves as a learning experience. An individual who worked on a project for years and has failed often would have a better experience than a person who has worked on it for three months. Always expect failure if you choose to grow, but make sure to learn from it. Failure is only a failure if you decide not to learn from it. You haven't failed until you quit.

Remember that failure is not the opposite of success; it is a path to success. The road to success is not a straight path. You would experience diverse challenges and obstacles, but they are an essential component to your success. Don't be afraid to fail. Don't see failure as failure. See failure as an opportunity for growth. Tony Robbins, a public speaker, life coach, author, and philanthropist, said this: "Have fun, be crazy, and be weird. Go out and screw up! You're going to anyway, so you may as well enjoy the process. Take the opportunity to learn from your mistakes: find the cause of your problems, and eliminate them. Don't try to be perfect; just be an excellent example of being human."

Rule Four
Put In the Hard Work

"Keep doing the hard things until the hard things become the easy things." – Unknown.

It was a sunny afternoon, I was chosen to participate in a school public speaking battle against three other students. Our supervisors gave each group three topics each for us to choose the one we are most comfortable with. After picking a topic, we were required to undergo school training to help build our public speaking skill, since that would be our first time. However, after the first day of training, I became tired of it. We were told we would need to learn how to confront our fear of speaking to large crowds of people, learn how to pause, eye contact, body language, and other needed skills. This was just too hard for me (it wasn't my thing at that time). So instead of building my craft bit-by-bit like the other two were, I decided to take the easy road. I barely attended the training and only focused more on content, rather than both content and delivery. To no one's surprise (except me), I failed terribly and became a laughing stock.

Whether you are preparing for a public presentation, or starting a new business, or becoming a father, or a mother, you'll have to understand that the only way for you to succeed at it is for you to put in the hard work. There's nothing great in life that didn't stem from hard work. Nothing spectacular comes without it. The Wright brothers, Bill Gates, Elon Musk, Thomas Edison, and Nikola Tesla are who they are because of the extra amount of effort they've put into their craft to become exceptional.

Colin Powell, former U.S. Defense Secretary, said, "A dream does not become reality through magic; it takes sweat, determination, and hard work." Companies that don't scout people with hard-working skills will only die in a short period. The interesting thing is, even though many of us are not the hard-working type, we tend to show more favouritism or hire people into our business that are more hard-working. This phenomenon is not only seen in businesses. It is widely known that the majority of smokers will prefer not to have a spouse that smokes. The majority of alcoholics will prefer not to also have their children being an alcoholic. We can also find this in our homes. Parents always want their children to achieve more than they (even when parents had the opportunity to be better).

Very few companies and individuals have ever failed when they applied hard work into their journey. One of the most important reasons for implementing hard work in your daily routine is to become exceptional. The only reason celebrities are celebrities, influencers are influencers, and why successful corporations are successful is because of the extra work they put into their routine compared to the majority. There's a very popular saying, "For you to have what you've never heard, you have to do what you've never done." That's it.

If you're tired of the life you are living, you feel like your family isn't where it's meant to be, your business isn't where you projected it, then, for all of those painful experiences to change for the better, you have to put in a better effort. We all demand great rewards, but we do very little to deserve them. Only those who put in the required efforts, that worked day-and-night, working their face-off to achieve greatness, are the people we remember as influencers and innovators. Hard work is hard work because only a few people can do it, and that's why it's really valuable for any company to have. The easy route leads to failure or at best, mediocrity. As Maria Bartiromo said, "Don't ever, ever, believe anyone who tells you that you can just by doing the easiest thing possible. Because there's always somebody behind you who wants to do what you're doing. And they're going to work harder than you if you're not working hard."

What about talent? Are they important?

When I ask people who they would prefer to work with: a person of hard work or a person of talent, most of the response I get is usually the latter. There's a common view that people with talent—who are gifted with brains to solve complex math or play sports effortlessly or any other skill with ease—are generally more successful than those who work day in, day out. However, is that verdict true? Before we dive in, let's look at what talent is.

Talent is a natural aptitude a person has in something. For example, a person could be good at singing with little or no training. You might have come across a talented person at school or at home (in fact, you might be one of them). These kinds of people are known to be gifted with a particular skill, meaning they tend to understand and implement certain skills quite easily than their peers.

Talents can come in different forms i.e., singing, sports, science, etc. People who are gifted with the abilities to solve complex mathematical equations do very little reading or studying for them to understand the equation quite well compared to their non-talented peers. Their peers could take hours or days before they could have the same level of understanding.

This attribute is one of the reasons why many hiring managers choose to hire people of great talent over hard-working individuals. According to an infographic from Davitt Corporate Partners, a firm specializing in business coaching and occupational psychology reveals that 60% of hiring managers would prefer to have talented people work for their company, even if it costs more. But that's not all. Another study conducted by the University College of London revealed participants were willing to relinquish even more to have a person of talent, including 8% in management skills, four years of leadership experience, and over $30,000 in accrued capital.

But if talent is more important than hard work, why is it that every top CEO, movie stars, sports stars, recognized authors, and other influencers always attribute their success to hard work.

"Work hard, have fun, make history." – Jeff Bezos, Amazon founder.

"I never took a day off in my 20s. Not one." – Bill Gates, Microsoft Co-founder.

"Talent is cheaper than table salt. What separates the talented individuals from the successful one is a lot of hard work." – Stephen King.

"Men die of boredom, psychological conflict, and disease. They do not die of hard work." – David Ogilvy, Advertising business tycoon.

"Hard work beats talent if talent doesn't work hard." – Tim Notke, Basketball Coach.

"Without labour, nothing prospers." – Sophocles, philosopher.

Anytime, any day, pure hard work will always defeat talent. We are living in a very competitive and fast-paced world that if a company relies purely on talent, such an entity could collapse. Talent alone can only carry one so far. However, to achieve greatness, one has to garner more skills to become better and improve their talent; if not, the talent will in no time prove to be worthless. Everyone is smart enough to have dreams, vision, or think of an innovative idea that could revolutionize the entire world, however, those ideals can only manifest if you put in the hard work.

Companies that are open to the mix of both talent and hard work stand the chance to achieve more. If you have both types of people in your business, you will not only achieve results but exceptional results. But you should encourage them both with hard work focused praise and talent-focused praise. For example:

Hard Work Focused Praise

- I notice and appreciate your hard efforts.
- You're such a hard worker
- I can tell you put a lot of work into this project.

Talent Focused Praise

- You are so smart.
- You are a prodigy.
- You are quick to assimilate.

You've got to understand that hard work is an essential primer for every success. The only way to the top is through hard work. However, when perfectly combined with talent, you produce a team that's almost impossible to beat. As Robert Griffin III said, "Hard work pays off. Hard work beats talent any day, but if you are talented and work hard, it's hard to beat."

What about working smart?

You've probably heard these words said to you, "don't work hard, work smart." Working smarts is a great thing to do—no doubt. It turns out that a lot of people waste tons of their time on activities that could be done with minimal effort. I read a story from a great book about how two friends, from the same village, thought of a way to earn some cash by helping the community to provide water to their home. Normally, the people that live in the community would have to go to the river, and then haul the water back to their home. So one of the two friends (who we will name, Frank) thought of easing the villagers' stress by helping them fetch the water himself and earn a little fee. Frank did this for months until his back fell off. The job was so onerous that he could hardly move the next day.

On the contrary, Frank's friend (who we will name, Joe) thought of a smart way of providing the villages with water very quickly. So what did he do? He decided to leave the village for a while in search of people who could provide him with some cash to build a small water distribution plant that would help supply all the villagers' constant stream of water for many years and collect some fee from them. So after Joe got the cash he needed from the investors, he built the plant and provided the villagers with all the water they would ever need, without Joe ever breaking a sweat.

I think you would agree that Joe worked smart. However, would you say Frank didn't work hard? In my opinion, I don't think Frank worked hard, rather, he worked dumb. We shouldn't confuse working hard with working dumb. So what does working dumb mean?

Good question. Working dumb can be seen as working hard on the wrong things or in the wrong way. It can be viewed as doing things right but never doing the right thing. Frank's approach was effective but nowhere efficient.

Joe's approach to achieving the result was both effective and efficient. But I also believe for you to work smart, you first have to work hard. I like to use a scenario of a man climbing a mountain to prove my point. If a man (or woman) attempts to climb mountain Everest for the very first time, it will always be harder than his second try, and his second try will be harder than his third try, and so on. It doesn't matter if the man worked smart on the first try, he will always get better in his second and subsequent attempts. And that's because of the amount of work he puts into each attempt. My point: The harder you work, the smarter you become.

Both hard work and smart work can't be separated. Every successful being that has ever walked on this planet (excluding those that inherited a possession) worked their butts off, each day, to become smarter and better at their skill. Don't confuse dumb work with hard work. The more you work hard, the smarter you become. To help buttress my point, here's a quote from Matshona Dhliwayo, a philosopher: "Work hard and you will earn good rewards. Work smart, and you will earn great rewards. Work hard and work smart, and you will earn extraordinary rewards." "Smart hard work" is what a friend of mine calls it.

Why hard work is so important

1. *Hard work gets results.* Working hard is always the baseline of great results. There's hardly ever a person who hasn't or wouldn't achieve results with hard work. It might take you days, months, or years before you get to achieve the result, but, eventually, it will occur. Do you want to earn more in your business? Do you want to get better grades? Is your relationship falling apart? Let me give an easy solution (but not simple) to those questions: Work more. Laziness doesn't amount to anything but wasted time and opportunities. Those who sit on their couch, hoping and praying for manna to come from heaven, or a white angel to bring them a Lamborghini, will wait till eternity. As Abraham Lincoln rightly said, "Things may come to those who wait, but only the things left by those who hustle." Do not exclude hard work in your toolkit for success.
2. *Hard work increases luck.* Yes, it does. When you work hard, you become more opportune to the favours of the world. The harder you work the luckier you become. Haven't you noticed this event yourself? The more you study for a school test or exam (say, SAT or ACT), the luckier you become at answering questions you just studied the other night. Those

who work hard find new opportunities always presenting themselves. Thomas Jefferson once said, "I'm a great believer in luck, and I find the harder I work, the more I have of it." So, if you want to attract more opportunities and increase your luck, work hard.

3. *Hard work builds character.* One of the best ways to develop the characters of leadership, discipline, and success is by working hard. The reason only a few people (compared to the rest of the world) become great leaders or create a multi-billion dollar company is because of their disciplined work ethic. Success isn't for the lazy or the wimps. Success isn't easy. Studies have shown that those who put in the time and extreme effort to body-build have a greater chance of succeeding and living a good life than those who care little about their health or do little to no exercise. Strong character is built the same way strong muscles are built—through hard work. It's easy to quit, however, quitting doesn't result in anything; instead, it paints a picture of a lack of discipline, commitment, and character. Don't be a quitter. Be a hard worker. It will pay you huge dividends for years to come.

Rule Five
Know When to Stop

Business doesn't fail because they don't know what to do; they fail because they don't know what to give up. — Peter Drucker.

Have you ever worked on a work project that later became very difficult but you weren't sure to quit or not? Or a friendship that became toxic, but you are not sure to continue the friendship or not? Everyone has experienced something like that. You are working on a task, you've spent all your time and resources on it, but you do not see the result you expected, and you are not sure whether to continue or not. Knowing when it's time to quit can be difficult, especially when you've been told words like this: "Winners never quit, and quitters never win."

However, there are times when you would need to face reality and accept that a plan just isn't working out and doesn't seem to in the future. Knowing when to stop is a vital skill to becoming successful and staying afloat. Many folks have experienced massive failures just because they were unable to stop and too persistent with their goals. Many companies have tanked just because they failed to challenge their thinking and be practical about their ambitions.

"It can be extremely exhausting to go back and forth in your mind, trying to decide whether it's time to quit something, and a lot of us dive into a pros and cons analysis in many areas of our lives, especially around big decisions... questioning whether you're dating their right person, should you move to a new city, end that friendship that's gotten super difficult, quit the job." Liz Traines, a life coach in Chicago.

"Depending on the time, energy, or financial investment you've made in the questioned area of your life, the harder it can be to determine what to do. It may not be something you can quantify on paper, and it can take time to evaluate your decision." She says.

Those who are unable to be practical about the ambition or goals and don't know the right time to take a step back are setting themselves up for a debacle. And when it comes to being practical about your life and the decisions you make, remember this: Sometimes there is no next time, no time-outs, and no second chances. Sometimes, it's now or never. When you quit something that drains you physically and mentally, you create room to spend your time doing things that bring you fulfilment and success. There are certain things you need to understand why many people fail to quit when the stats show it.

Sunk Cost Fallacy

A sunk cost is the cost that has already been paid for and cannot be recovered. The sunk cost effect is the tendency for people to continue an endeavour or continue consuming or pursuing an option if they've invested time, money, or other resources to it. The sunk cost fallacy is when a person or company sticks with a decision because they've already put the money down for it and want to make sure it isn't lost. For example, a person may have a $20 ticket to a concert and then drive for hours through a blizzard, just because he feels the impulse to attend due to having made the initial investments. Similarly, if a person goes to a restaurant and becomes full after eating half of the meal, he/she is forced to over-eat so that the money doesn't get wasted.

The sunk cost effect often happens in relationships. A classic example of sunk cost fallacy: In a relationship, the longer you've been together, the harder it is to break up: "I've invested a lot in the relationship, it would be stupid of me to quit now." In *The Art of Thinking Clearly*, Rolf Dobelli wrote this: The sunk cost fallacy is most dangerous when we have invested a lot of time, money, energy, or love in something. This investment becomes a reason to carry on, even if we are dealing with a lost cause. The more we invest, the higher the sunk cost is, and the greater the urge to continue becomes.

"But I do think people do these things because they want to convince themselves that they've managed to recapture the loss," Christopher Olivola, an assistant professor of marketing at Carnegie Mellon's Tepper School of Business said. "Or it could be an attempt to convince others and ourselves that we're not wasteful." It is an irrational act since the money, love, and energy invested can't be recovered—a sunk cost.

Be practical about your decisions. What's done is done. Instead of pursuing things that make you feel drained of resources, or that makes you worse off, focus and invest in things that are working. Go into a new relationship if the one you're in doesn't make you feel good and happy. If you've paid for a class that has been useless to you, stop it. If you're one hour into a movie already, but the film doesn't interest you, stop it and watch an exciting film.

Loss Aversion

Loss aversion is the behavioural tendency for people to prefer to avoid losses compared to gaining the equivalent amount. This behaviour is at work when we make decisions and choices that include both the possibility of a loss or gain. For example, losing $300 would cost you a higher amount of happiness than the delight you would feel if you received the same amount. It means you would experience more pain when you lose a property. You may, however, feel a slight delight if you were to be giving the same thing. Recent studies have shown that a loss "weighs" about twice that of a similar gain.

Behavioural science expert, Amos Tversky and Daniel Kahneman performed an experiment that resulted in a clear example of human bias towards losses. The research involved asking people if they would accept a bet based on the flip of a coin. If the coin came up heads, the individual would lose $100, but if it flipped tails, he/she wins $200. The result of the experiment showed that, on average, people needed twice as much as they were willing to lose to proceed forward with the bet.

Loss aversion is an evolutionary act. When confronted with a predator during a hunt for food or searching for new territory, our primordial ancestors would prefer avoiding the beast with the possibility of losing the food they've gathered to avoid being maimed, lose a tribe member, or even worse—their life. It is our nature. However, loss aversion is not always unfortunate, as in many cases, it is beneficial to our way of life. Our ancestors were able to survive because of their instinct to not lose: children, or their life. In the business world, it helps us shy away from investments or decisions that are potentially harmful to our business.

One of the reasons for loss aversion is attachments to objects. When we are attached or form a secure connection to something or someone, it becomes hard to let go. Supposing your mom gave you a necklace that's worth $50, you may feel uncomfortable selling it, even if someone offered you a higher amount, say $100.

Loss aversion played a role in the refusal of Yahoo to be sold to Microsoft for $44.6 billion in 2008. Jerry Yang and David Filo were the founders of Yahoo. Yang was, at the time, Yahoo's CEO. Their attachment to the company, perhaps, made the founders make a lousy decision on refusing the offer of Microsoft. Despite their steady decline of value, as they were overshadowed by Google (which they failed to buy for a mere $1 million in 1997 and once again in 2002), they decided not to sell, which later cost them a lot. In a letter to Yang, Steve Ballmer, former Microsoft CEO, suggested that Yahoo would live to regret its defiance, insisting that the firm had "left significant value on the table." Google's parent company, Alphabet, is now the third US tech company worth $1 trillion.

Loss aversion is the reason why they sold the company for $4.6 billion to Verizon in 2016. When they noticed that their market value had shrunk significantly, their primitive instinct not to lose kicked in, they were losing market valuation year after year. The point is: Be practical about your decisions.

Overconfidence Bias

This is one of the most significant cognitive biases. Overconfidence can cause you to experience problems because you may not have adequately prepared for the situation. Overconfidence bias is the propensity to over-estimate your abilities and talent. Your overconfidence gives you a false assumption that you are better than others due to the hyper-inflated sense of your intellect, skills, or self-belief. We tend to think we know more than we actually do. Eighty-two percent of US drivers consider themselves to be in the top thirty percent of their group in terms of safety. Eighty-one percent of new business owners felt they had an excellent chance of their business succeeding. When asked about the success of their peers, they answered thirty-nine percent.

A large proportion of newlyweds believe their marriage will endure when asked just right before their wedding night. You are most likely not as smart as you might think. Eighty-seven percent of MBA students at Stanford rated their academic performance as above the median. Sixty-five percent of Americans consider themselves above average in intelligence.

The thing is, you can easily spot overconfidence in others but not your own. Many of us go into business with little or no information about it. Yet, we invest a lot into it, believing we would succeed. That's overconfidence.

Examples of overconfidence

1. "Heavier-than-air flying machines are impossible." – Lord Kelvin, British mathematician, 1895.
2. "Man will never reach the moon, regardless of all future scientific advances." – Lee Deforest, inventor of the vacuum tube, 1957.
3. "There is no reason for anyone to have a computer in their home." – Ken Olson, President of Digital Equipment Company, 1977.

Now that you've understood some of the cognitive biases that may skew your decision-making process. You need to ask yourself questions that would create a rational explanation for your choice.

1. Is my business, goal, or relationship still progressing? Before you quit on anything—relationship, job, business, or goal, it is critical to know if there have been any continuous improvements. Yahoo would have probably sold the company earlier if it had noticed its decline in market value. You must always be aware of the state of your investment. If there's continuous growth, keep it. If there is a steady or rapid decline, renovate or better still, jump ship. Ask yourself this: "What real-world data or statistics do I have to verify that this business, relationship, or goal is progressing week after week, month after month, or year after year?" Once you've determined the presence of augmentation, you then ask...

2. Is it still fulfilling and fun? Tony Robbins had an interview with Darren Hardy, author of *Compound Effect*. In it, Tony said: "I have seen many business moguls achieve their ultimate goals but still live in frustration, worry, and fear. So what's depriving many business magnates of being fulfilled? The problem is, they've set a priority for accomplishments over fulfilment and happiness." Immense achievements and awards don't guarantee a sense of purpose and can't replace the need for fulfilment. It doesn't matter how valuable or successful your company is; if you are not having fun or being fulfilled, it is worthless. Tony Robbins spoke these words: "The art of fulfilment is the ability to experience the thrill of the chase, and the magic of the moment, the unbridled joy of feeling truly alive." Of course, the definition of fulfilment and fun is different for all of us. Still, if you invest your resources on something or someone that makes you feel awful or worse off at the end of the day, there's no point in continuing. Your resources should be invested in a path that is fulfilling to you. Ask yourself this: Does my goal keep me excited each day? Am I waking up thrilled to go to work every morning? Do I long to spend more time and create an unforgettable experience with

my partner? Does my business make me fulfilled despite the success?

So, the question is: When should you quit?

When you are not able to give a YES to both questions. When your business, relationship, job, or goals aren't progressing, and when you don't find it satisfying and fulfilling to keep on doing it. Commit these words to mind: *Success without fulfilment is a failure.* You now have the blueprint to help guide your decisions as you evaluate your 9-5 job, business, and relationship. Quitting something you've spent energy, time, money, and developed an emotional attachment to is never going to be easy; however, how you assess whether it's time to quit or not doesn't have to be complicated.

9

Principle #9: Develop A Willful Mind

Grit is living life like it's a marathon, not a sprint. — Angela Duckworth.

Have you ever set goals that you later realized was just too hard to accomplish? Everyone understands the importance of intelligence quotient (IQ) and talent for success. But, only a few people necessarily understand and apply grit in their lives. Grit is an essential factor that affects your ability to achieve long-term goals. Angela Duckworth, a world's leading expert on grit and author of *Grit: The Power of Passion and Perseverance*, explains grit as the passion and sustained persistence applied toward long-term achievement, with no particular concern for rewards or recognition along the way. In simpler terms, it's the ability to persevere and be passionate about a long-term goal, even when you face obstacles.

Many of the success achieved by successful people and big corporations is because of their grit. Grit gives you the physiological and mental fuel to push on, even when it seems challenging. Grit allows you to say, "I will do this, no matter what." "I will not stop until I win." The Apollo 11 spaceflight mission to the moon happened with the help of grit. Before the spaceflight to the moon, it took years of trying, testing, and failing. The United States was pressured by the Soviet Union to achieve the first spaceflight to the moon, known as the Space Race. Without the mix of grit into their chase, the U.S. wouldn't have been the first. Talent isn't enough. Knowledge isn't enough. You need persistence and passion for the pursuit of goals that could take months, years, or even decades to achieve. The level of passion and persistence I have for writing and technology has pushed me to greater heights. Not talent.

Grit is a skill and mindset that can be developed over time. It permits you to stand up to any challenges with self-control and believe that you can be victorious amid obstacles. It gives you the persistence to finish what you've started, especially when it matters to you. People who have mastered the power of grit don't belittle their abilities and can set tough goals with the mindset of achieving them no matter how long it takes. You've heard of Thomas Edison and how he was able to invent the electric light-bulb even after failing many times. He was widely known for his persistence and passion for his projects, known to never give up on things. He wasn't afraid to make mistakes. He famously said, "I have not failed. I've just found 10,000 ways that won't work."

Edison's intelligence wasn't the cause of his success. When he was a child, he was thought to be dumb and told that he would never succeed by many of his "intelligent" teachers. His grit (passion and perseverance) was the cause of his significant achievements, not intellect. People with grit have an I-must-succeed-no-matter-what attitude that makes them successful.

People with grit are never afraid to fail, never afraid to set higher goals, never scared to try something new—to take a new path. They always surpass people's expectations. That's why grit is a necessary trait to have that makes you succeed in business and life. Steve Jobs's passion for innovation made him stood out from the crowd of tinkerers, even though his intellect and skills may not be exceptional compared to his peers. In an interview with Bill Gates, Jobs said: "People say you've to have a lot of passion for what you're doing, and it's totally true. The reason is, that, it's so hard that, if you don't, any rational person would give up."

In 2007, Angela Duckworth published a paper about grit in the Journal of Personality and Social Psychology, showing that grit was an essential predictor of accomplishment. In a longitudinal study of more than 11,000 West Point cadets, Duckworth says, "I was looking for a context in which people might be quitting too early. There's such a thing as quitting at the right time. But there's also such a thing as quitting on a bad day when you're discouraged and maybe shouldn't be making such a big decision." After an extensive two-year process, each cadet who enters West Point must finish a six-week initiation nicknamed Beast Barracks during the summer preceding classes.

The report showed that, on average, three out of every one hundred cadets dropped out during this training. Duckworth realized that during Beast Barrack training, grit was crucial. "The grittier you are, the less likely you are to drop out during that very discouraging time," Duckworth explains.

Equation for Achievement

You need more than just talent and skill to succeed in a competitive world. It takes effort.

Duckworth's equation for achievement:

Talent **X** Effort = Skill

Skill **X** Effort = Achievement

"Talent is how quickly your skills improve when you invest effort. Achievement is what happens when you take your acquired skills and use them." Duckworth explained. Thomas Edison, Steve Jobs, and others wouldn't have achieved historical results if it weren't for their effort. Without effort, even the smartest, most skilled, most gifted in the world will not accomplish much. People with grit understands that challenges and obstacles are a normal part of life, and to get the most out of it, they have to be gritty each day. They understand that a more significant challenge doesn't imply defeat; instead, it means more excellent opportunity for growth.

The Brain of a Gritty Mind

Note: This is an oversimplified explanation of how the brain improves memory and skill.

The brain is just like a muscle; if it's not being used, it will waste away. It consists of billions of nerve cells called neurons. Each neuron is connected to other neurons through synapses, sites where signals are transmitted in the form of chemical messengers that allows the neurons to communicate. Just like the muscle, if the brain is not used, it will lose its abilities.

When you spend lots of time exercising and lifting weights, your muscles will grow (muscle hypertrophy). But when you stop exercising, you will experience loss of skeletal muscle (muscle atrophy). The brain needs constant exercise, which it gets when you work hard and learn new skills. When you do these things, your brain undergoes what is called *neuroplasticity.*

Neuroplasticity is the brain's ability to reorganize itself by forming new neural connections. Challenging the brain by learning new skills and putting extra effort into an activity changes the brain as it creates and strengthens the neural connections that are needed to grow, and removes the neural connections it doesn't need. The reason why we improve our skills when we put in efforts daily is that the brain forms the right neural pathway that enhances our ability. When you stop practising, your performance level begins to depreciate as the connection of neurons weakens. If you stress the brain with consistent training and practice, you'll develop the mental toughness to handle stressful situations and keep going. The brain is less able to change when you become an adult, making it more challenging to learn new skills. Children can learn faster than adults because of the development of their brains until adolescents. Improved memory or skill isn't about having increased brain volume but having a strong network of neurons.

Here are some of the things you could do to strengthen your brain:

- Build things
- Try using your non-dominant hand
- Pick up a new hobby
- Eat healthy and exercise
- Read books
- Build your vocabulary
- Learn a new language
- Use the skills you've already gained frequently

As we try new things and put in the daily effort, the brain goes to develop that skill. The more you stress your brain with hard work, the more connections your brain will create. James Loehr, an expert on peak performance, says, "Stress (in moderation) is not the enemy in our life; paradoxically, it's the key to growth." Always make sure to push yourself harder. And remember: Your brain will only grow and be strengthened if you put it to work. Live the advice of Bill Gates: "Surround yourself with people who challenge you, teach you, and push you to be your best self."

Intelligent Quotient Vs. Grit

By the Oxford Dictionary, intelligence is the ability to acquire and apply knowledge and skills. Intelligence quotient (IQ) is a measure of a person's reasoning ability. It is supposed to help evaluate how well someone can use information and logic to solve problems, answer questions, or make predictions. The IQ test has been used to help identify students who would do well in fast-paced "gifted education" programs. Even the U.S. government and its military use IQ test to choose who to hire. These IQ tests help predicts who will make a good leader or be better at specific skills. The IQ test has been used in companies to "accurately" predict a job candidate's future performance. Bill Gates once said in an interview, "The key for us, number one, has always been hiring brilliant people. There is no way of getting around that in terms of IQ, you've got to be very elitist in picking the people who deserve to write software." Gates was talking specifically about Microsoft; however, there has been a great deal of research suggesting that general cognitive ability may be a good predictor of job performance and success in life.

The importance of IQ in evaluating how well you're going to perform at the workplace is crucial. In 2014, Adam Grant, a Wharton psychologist, published a post on LinkedIn arguing that emotional intelligence (EQ), a term brought to fashion by Daniel Goleman, an author of *Emotional Intelligence*, describes the ability to identify and manage your own emotions and others, is less important than cognitive ability (the capacity to learn) when it comes to job performance.

According to studies Grant conducted on hundreds of salespeople and hundreds of applicants for sales positions, Grant concluded: "Cognitive ability was more than five times more powerful than emotional intelligence. The average employee with high cognitive ability generated annual revenue of over $195,000 compared with $159,000 for those with moderate cognitive ability and $109,000 for those with low cognitive ability. Emotional intelligence added nothing after measuring cognitive ability." In Joseph and Newman's comprehensive analysis, cognitive ability accounted for more than fourteen percent of job performance. Emotional intelligence accounted for less than one percent.

Anyone can be angry—that is easy. But to be angry with the right person, to the right degree, at the right time, for the right purpose and in the right way—that is not easy. — Aristotle.

Does it mean emotional intelligence is useless? Of course not! "It's relevant to performance in jobs where you have to deal with emotions every day like sales, real estate, and counselling," Grant explains. If you are helping people manage their emotions, it can be of great use to understand your team's feelings and respond appropriately. But in professions like engineering, accounting, or science that lack these emotional needs, EQ didn't account for better performance. If your job is to repair a car or work in a melting plant, paying attention to emotions might distract you from working efficiently and effectively.

In 2016, Kashmea Wahi, an 11-year-old Indian-origin girl in London, achieved the top possible score of 162 on an IQ test of Mensa—the international test that gauges the IQ, becoming one of the youngest brainiest students in the country. Her IQ score beats Albert Einstein's score. On an IQ test, a score of 100 is average; someone who scores 125 or above is in the top five percent. The two most common IQ tests are the Wechsler scales and the Stanford-Binet intelligence scale. Individual variations of these are now used by the military, some schools, the National Football League, and employers.

It is tempting to infer that a high IQ score is a critical component of success, if not the only one. Most people think intelligence is the reason why successful people do so well. Psychologists who study intelligence find this to be partly right. It takes a lot more than intelligence to achieve success. Intelligence matters, but not as much as you might think.

Let's talk about Grit

Stephen Hawking was regarded as one of the most brilliant theoretical physicists in history. He won various awards—Copley Medal, Albert Einstein Award, Wolf Prize in Physics, Audie Award for Science Fiction, Hughes Medal, James Clerk Maxwell Medal and Prize, and many more. But his intelligence wasn't the real cause of his success and the reason he lived longer than his doctor expected.

Stephen Hawking was born in England on January 8, 1942—three hundred years to the day after the death of, the astronomer, Galileo Galilei. In early 1963, just shy of his 21st birthday, Hawking was diagnosed with Amyotrophic Lateral Sclerosis (ALS). It is a motor neuron disease that stopped his muscles from working, implying that he could not walk, talk, raise his hands, and other parts of his body. He was not expected to live for more than two years. As the disease spreads, Hawking became less mobile and began using a wheelchair. He lost his speech and the ability to move his hands. Yet, Hawking defied the odds, not only attaining his PhD and contributing significantly to the scientific community but also living long enough to seventy-six, after living with the disease for fifty-five years.

He died on March 14, 2018.

The reason for Hawking's success wasn't his intelligence, but his passion for science and the perseverance he had, and perhaps, made him lived longer than expected. Even with his disabilities, he became a famous writer that went on to write lots of nonfiction books. His first book, *A Brief History of Time*, was first published in 1988 and became an international bestseller. In it, Hawking aimed to communicate questions about the birth and death of the universe to the layperson. His other books include: *The Universe in a Nutshell, The Grand Design,* and *On the Shoulders of Giants.*

What do Oprah Winfrey, Michael Jordan, Walk Disney, J.K. Rowlings, and Martin Luther King have in common? They are passionate and persistent. You might have seen a long time schoolmate who, at the time, was the genius with the highest IQ in class. All the teacher thought he would be a bright inventor or a successful person but later turned out not to be the case. Many smart and intelligent people in the world can do quick, complex multiplications to solve complex puzzles but are still unable to achieve great success. It turns out that intelligence isn't a key predictor of future success.

Duckworth has spent years researching and studying people, trying to understand what makes high achievers successful. But what she found surprised her. It wasn't SAT scores. It wasn't IQ scores. It wasn't even a degree from Ivy League schools that turned out to be the critical predictor of success. Grit was. Hawking's passion and burning desire pushed him to live longer. Use your passion, perseverance, drive, or grit to achieve success and live a happy life.

"It was this combination of passion and perseverance that made high achievers special," Duckworth said. "In a word, they had grit." It doesn't matter how intelligent you are; if you aren't passionate about your goals and can't persevere, you will fail. You have to develop the will to keep on learning, keep on growing, and keep on pushing back until your goals are realized. Being gritty is vital to your success. It's about always pushing yourself and being driven to excel. Duckworth found that, for highly successful people, being passionate about their dreams and goals is an important character. Even if some of the things they had to do were annoying, frustrating, or painful, they wouldn't dream of giving up. Their passion was enduring. Your intelligence doesn't matter. Your talent doesn't matter. What matters is your passion and perseverance—your grit.

Duckworth's research shows that to succeed or achieve great things, you don't have to be the smartest person in the class or the most intelligent person in your workplace. That is not important. What matters most is the effort you exhaust toward your goals and your logical drive throughout your career.

I failed in some subjects in exam, but my friend passed in all. Now he is an engineer in Microsoft, and I am the owner of Microsoft. — *Bill Gates*

Is grit a better predictor of future success than IQ? Based on studies and research, Yes. Intelligence is an important skill to have to achieve success. But the significance of intelligence is boldly recognized in only a few fields such as science, engineering, and information technology. Contrary, grit is a skill that is very important in all forms of fields and life. A weight lifter relies heavily on grit to succeed rather than intelligence. To run a 26.2 miles marathon doesn't require you being smart; instead, it requires a great deal of training, stamina, and an extreme will to win.

You don't need to be smart to be a great comedian, an actor, an athlete, a singer, a pilot, a soldier, a preacher, an activist, or an engineer. You don't even need to be a genius to become a great physicist. What you need most is the passion for your work and the dedication to keep on growing in rough and smooth times. You can only achieve little with talent alone. You can only achieve little with intelligence alone. With grit, you can achieve high success. From this time forth, I urge you to always include grit in your formula for success.

Grit, as you now appreciate, is a required skill to become a high achiever. But there's also another skill all successful people have in their lives: Delayed Gratification.

Delayed Gratification

In the 1960s, Walter Mischel, a psychologist and Stanford professor, ex-perimented on a group of four-year-olds. The experiment was made to understand the importance of self-control and delayed gratification and how they can have an essential trait for success in their personal and professional life. The experiment was called *The Marshmallow Experiment.* The experiment began by bringing each child into a room, sitting them down in a chair, and presented them with various treats, including marshmallows.

The researcher offered a deal to the kids. The researcher told the kids that after he leaves the room, they could eat one marshmallow right away, or if they could wait for a few minutes, they could eat two marshmallows. The choice was: one marshmallow right now or two marshmallows later. The researcher left the room for a few minutes. This was what they noticed: Some of the kids were unable to control their desire to eat the marshmallow just after the researcher left. Only a few (about thirty percent) of the kids managed to control their urge to eat the marshmallow and received double their treats when the researcher came back fifteen minutes later.

Years later, the researchers conducted follow up studies on the kids and tracked each child's progress in several areas. By now, the kids were much grown. What the researchers found was surprising. The researchers asked about their grades and SAT scores, the ability to develop social skills, how they handled problems, and their capacity to cope with stress. They found that those four-year-old kids who delayed gratification longer became more cognitively and socially competent adolescents, achieving higher academic performance. They coped better with frustration and stress. They were more accessible and involved themselves in fewer drugs. They developed practical self-regulatory skills early that gave them an advantage throughout their lives. The children who were able to wait longer during the experiment later were more rational, verbally fluent, and planed better. In other words, this series of experiments proved that the ability to delay gratification was crucial for success in life.

Because of our biology, we humans tend to move to the path of the least pain. Avoiding temptations that are standing right in front of us so that we can hold out for something substantially better down the line—for many of us, that's a battle we struggle to win. Rather than choosing the steep path of delaying pleasure for a bigger purpose, we tend to seek out things that would give us instant results with less pain. For example:

1. Instead of exercising regularly to reduce body fat, people prefer going for liposuction (a surgical procedure that uses suction techniques to remove fat) to get the desired shape—that's if they try to reduce fat at all.
2. Instead of finding or creating a job to earn money, people would prefer

to spend their money in casinos, hoping to get rich quickly.

3. Instead of eating healthy foods (fruits and vegetables), people prefer to take dietary supplements and certain medications to live longer.

Successful people would not have achieved their success if it weren't for their ability to delay gratification. Achieving success is not an easy or painless task. You would have to sacrifice a lot of things: alcohol, TV, and lavish spending. You would have to quit on activities you normally relish when working towards your goal. If you delay the gratification of spending lavishly, then you'll be able to save more for the raining days—or else, you'll get drenched. If you delay the pleasure of watching television and focus more on your homework or project, you'll get better grades and complete your project. If you delay the gratification of playing too much and spend less time with an unproductive friend, you'll achieve more in a shorter time. Success usually comes down to choosing the pain of discipline over pleasure. And that's what delayed gratification is all about.

The obsession with instant gratification blinds us from our long-term potential. — Mike Dooley

If the ability to delay gratification is an essential trait to succeed, then why isn't everyone doing it?

Many folks are often inclined to pursue short-term rewards because the payoffs are closer to see and more comfortable to attain than making the arduous effort to attain long-term rewards. Do you know: Jeff Bezos didn't make any profit for over five years while running Amazon, all for a bigger future reward? Delayed gratification is always laborious because the reward is in the distant future and uncertain. Delaying the satisfaction of having an ice-cream right now for the future reward of reducing weight, doesn't feel like an excellent choice. Delaying the satisfaction of having to eat a burger right now for the possibility of not being obese, doesn't feel worth it at that moment.

Avoiding instant gratification for a future reward looks like this: You choose to accept a $1000 cash a year from now, instead of a $100 cash right now. But if the person dies before a full year, you won't get the money.

This uncertainty makes giving up immediate rewards so complicated and tricky, unlike the kids in Mischel's experiment who had the certainty of receiving the second marshmallow if they should delay their urge to eat the marshmallow immediately. However, the real world doesn't always come with this guarantee. You might choose to quit eating sugary and fatty foods, but still became obese or die prematurely. There's no certainty.

In an article in Cognition, Joseph W. Kable, and Joseph J. McGuire, neuro-scientists from the University of Pennsylvania suggest that our uncertainty about distant rewards is the main reason why delaying satisfaction is so brutal. "The timing of the real-world event is not always so predictable," they explain. "Decision-makers routinely wait for buses, job offers, weight loss, and other outcomes characterized by significant temporal uncertainty." Not knowing when or if your long-term reward—longevity, a good job, or $1000—will ever arrive, is the rationale why many people fail to discipline themselves. However, despite the fact that delaying gratification is ultimately the best path, deciding to choose instant pleasure might not always be a wrong decision.

In a bet, a person that decides to stop at earning $3000 rather than continuing playing with the possibility of winning $5000 or losing it all, probably made the right call. In casinos, many people lose money because of their "I will win more money if I could just keep on playing" believe. They fail to stop at their little wins, but they continue playing, hoping to win "big" in a few minute or hour. Kable and McGuire suggest, "While going for the immediate reward is often viewed as a loss of self-control and giving in to temptation, it can represent a rational action in cases where a promised reward is uncertain or unlikely."

How to improve your ability to delay gratification

The ability to delay gratification is a skill that can be improved and learned. Here are some of the various ways to enhance your ability to wait.

1. *Break your long-term goals into short-term goals.* It is not easy to visualize long-term goals and invest the effort to work towards them. When things are far from us, we become discouraged from hunting for them. However, if you can bring your long-term goals close enough to visualize and within your reach, that would motivate and energize you to pursue your goals. Break your goals into smaller ones. If your goal is to write a book within a year, break it down into months or weeks. Instead of focusing on completing your book within a year, which could discourage you from starting in the first place, preferably, emphasis on finishing a chapter within a month, which is much closer than a year. When you can break a long-term goal into a short-term goal, you'll become motivated to start and finish the journey of achieving your goal.

2. *Set realistic deadlines.* Being practical about your deadlines is very crucial to your success. When trying to set a goal, people tend to underestimate the time it will take to achieve their goals because of our desire to have things quickly. For instance, setting a goal to write a book of over three hundred pages that is well organized and informative within a month, isn't a realistic deadline. When the person isn't able to achieve his or her goal within that deadline, he or she becomes discouraged and gives in to the temptation of watching Netflix all day. A realistic goal of thirty pages a week would allow such a person to see results and be encouraged to continue writing more pages. Most people overestimate what they can do in a year and underestimate what they can achieve in five years.

3. *Reward yourself.* Achieving goals might not be a fun process, but the reward you get can make it worthwhile. When you set goals for yourself, always make sure to reward yourself in-between. If your goal is to lose a pound per week and you achieve it, reward yourself with activities you would typically enjoy doing: Spend time with friends or even take a

day break to recoup your energy and motivation. When you anticipate a reward just before you complete a goal, it motivates and pushes you to finish what you have started. It is a powerful way of making a habit, also. For those who have goals to lose weight, during this reward period, make sure not to reward yourself with items that increase your weight, such as sugary beverages, cakes, and fatty foods.

Those who can delay instant gratification for a better future reward are those who are patient. Steve Jobs didn't reach his level of fame within a day. Jeff Bezos didn't become the richest man in the world overnight. Michael Jordan didn't become one of the world's best athletes with just a day of training. The most significant scientific discoveries didn't take a day's work for it to be realized. All great things in life are achieved with patience. If you are not able to develop the skill of patience, you won't be able to delay satisfaction, therefore, you won't be able to make much in life.

Researchers have found that people who put off their instant urge for something they believe in, often succeed in life. Success requires heart-and-soul effort, and you can put your heart and soul only into something you believe. It may take months, years, or even decades to reach your long-term goals. However, those willing to put in the effort (passion and perseverance) and the ability to delay immediate gratification will enjoy a better professional and personal life. As Brian Tracy puts it, "The ability to discipline yourself to delay gratification in the short term in order to enjoy greater rewards in the long term is the indispensable prerequisite for success."

Author's Note

We've come to the end of the book. If you read or listened to all nine principles, I thank and congratulate you on the committed journey you embarked on. But here are a few things that I would love you to do.

First, take a picture of you reading this book and share it on Instagram, Facebook, or Twitter and tag it with "I am now a #HighAchiever." This activity helps me to know where you're reading this from and I'll love to see where you at.

Second, it is not just enough to listen or read a personal development book, you also have to implement each principle, and put in the work to get high achieving results that you desire. If knowledge were the only criteria for success, then anyone with access to the internet would be successful. But that's not the case.

I know from experience that the principles I have shared with you will work immensely in your life if you diligently apply them. Nothing changes just because you read a book. It's what you do with the knowledge you've gained that would result in change. If you feel the need to reread this book, then I suggest you do so and apply the principles and bits of knowledge that is presented in the book until you're using them effectively in every area of your life. There is nothing more wasteful than spending hours of your time watching a show, listening, or reading a book without getting valuable and practical results at the end of it.

The principles won't be easy to implement at first, but you know by now that success takes time. Becoming a high achiever isn't going to be easy or come overnight. Stick with the principles, and over time it will pay you huge dividends.

So I want to thank you again for reading this book, and please do share it with a friend, coworker, relative, or stranger. Helping someone else become better is an act of mentorship and a trait all high achievers embody. Sharing this book to others could not just change their lives, but their generation to come. As you already know, help doesn't just make the recipient feel better, but it also makes you feel great. Bill Gates, Warren Buffett, and Tony Robbins do philanthropy for the same reason because they understand the ripple effect of helping others.

My goal is to help people become more than their current selves. By sharing this book, you are helping in making my goal a reality. And it will also make the world more prosperous.

Also, please do remember to leave a review for this book on Amazon, Bookbub, or Goodreads. Your review goes a long way in fostering my writing career and you can help personally by leaving an honest review. The review can be a line or two.

It goes a long way in motivating others, as well, to get a copy of their own. Your reviews will be read by me and taken into thought so as to make my next book much valuable and exciting for you.

With that said, thank you for joining me on this incredible voyage to help make a difference in the life of others. Until next time, have a fulfilling life.

Thanks,

Alfred Ayokunle.

Connect With Me

Do you have questions that you need help with concerning what you've read or to get a direct update on any future developments?

You can reach me at the social links listed below.

- Facebook Author Page: https://www.fb.me/alfredayokunle
- Twitter: @ayokunlealfred
- Instagram: @ayokunlealfred
- Bookbub: https://www.bookbub.com/authors/alfred-ayokunle
- Goodreads: https://www.goodreads.com/author/show/20955520.Alfred_Ayokunle

Acknowledgement

This book wouldn't have been completed without the assistance and guidance of some tremendous people. Thanks to my parents who helped me with proofreading the draft. Though I didn't inform my parents (including my close friends) about this book when I was writing it, when I was done I finally opened it to my parents and friends and they were happy and willing to help in any way they could.

Finally, to all those who read this book and commits to pass it on to someone else (either friend or foe), I want to say Thank You!

It's important for everyone to begin to understand and appreciate the importance of their health and how to develop themselves to become great leaders and achieve a big success in life.

Being a HIGH ACHIEVER should be your priority because that's who you are created to be. Writing this book has been an incredible journey, and thank you for being on the ride with me.

Recommended Books

When: The scientific secrets of perfect timing by Daniel H. Pink

Why We Sleep: Unlocking the power of sleep and dreams by Matthew Walker

The Story of the Human Body: Evolution, Health, and Disease by Daniel Lieberman

The Power of Habit: Why we do what we do in life and business by Charles Duhigg

The Ride of a Lifetime: Lessons learned from 15 years of CEO of the Walt Disney Company by Robert Iger

The Molecule of More by Daniel Z. Lieberman

Unlock It: The Master Key to Wealth, Success, and Significance by Dan Lok

The making of a manager: What to do when everyone looks to you by Julie Zhuo

The Lean Startup by Eric Ries

The Magic of Thinking Big by David J Schwartz

The Art of Thinking Clearly by Rolf Dobelli

Start With Why: How great leaders inspire everyone to take action by Simon Sinek

Misbehaving: The making of behavioral economics by Richard H. Thaler

Just Listen: Discover the secret to getting through to absolutely anyone by Mark Goulston

Grit: The power of passion and perseverance by Angela Duckworth

Man's Search For Meaning by Victor E. Frankl

Give and Take by Adam Grant

Contagious: Why things catch on by Jonah Berger

Deep Work: Rules for focused success in a distracted world by Cal Newport

The Velvet Rope Economy: How inequality became big business by Nelson

D. Schwartz

Can't Hurt Me: Master your mind and defy the odds by David Goggins

CashFlow Quadrant: Guide to financial freedom by Robert Kiyosaki

Creativity: Overcoming the unseen forces that stand in the way of true inspiration by Ed Catmull

Emotional First Aid by Guy Winch

Extreme Ownership: How U.S. Navy SEALs Lead and Win by Jocko Willink

The Book of Joy by Dalai Lama

Sources

Principle #1

Javanbakht, A. J., & Saab, L.S. *What Happens in the Brain When We Feel Fear: And why some of us just can't get enough of it.* SMITHSONIANMAG.com. October 27, 2017. https://www.smithsonianmag.com/science-nature/what-happens-brain-feel-fear-180966992/.

Schwartz, T. S. *Why Fear Kills Productivity.* NYT. December 5, 2014. https://dealbook.nytimes.com/2014/12/05/reduce-fear-to-create-a-calmer-productive-workplace/.

Heathfield, S. M. *Understanding Stress and How It Affects Your Workplace Woman sitting at table speaking during a conference call: If You Know What Cause Stress, You Can Manage It for Well-Being.* TheBalanceCareers.com. May 4, 2020. https://www.thebalancecareers.com/understanding-stress-and-how-it-affects-the-workplace-1919200.

Lindberg, S. L. *Psychological Stress.* Healthline.com. February 1, 2019. https://www.healthline.com/health/psychological-stress#good-and-bad.

Betty-Ann Heggie. *The Benefits of Laughing in the Office.* HBR.org. November 16, 2018. https://www.google.com/amp/s/hbr.org/amp/2018/11/the-benefits-of-laughing-in-the-office

Principle #2

Abrams, A. A. *Overcoming the Need to Please: Stop trying so hard to get others to like you, and start liking yourself.* Psychology Today. October 1, 2017. https://www.google.com/amp/s/www.psychologyto-day.com/us/blog/nurturing-self-compassion/201710/overcoming-the-need-please%3famp.

Renken, E. R. *Most Americans Are Lonely, And Our Workplace Culture May Not*

Be Helping. NPR.org. January 23, 2020. https://www.npr.org/sections/health-shots/2020/01/23/798676465/most-americans-are-lonely-and-our-workplace-culture-may-not-be-helping

Centers for Disease Control and Prevention. 2020. *Loneliness and Social Isolation Linked to Serious Health Conditions.* https://www.cdc.gov/aging/publications/features/lonely-older-adults.html.

Shaw, G.S. *9 subtle signs that you're lonely — even if it doesn't feel like it.* INSIDER. October 9, 2018. https://www.insider.com/signs-of-loneliness-2018-6

Louise C. Hawkley, Ph.D. and John T. Cacioppo, Ph.D. 2010. *Loneliness Matters: A Theoretical and Empirical Review of Consequences and Mechanisms.* NCBI. https://www.ncbi.nlm.nih.gov/pmc/articles/PMC3874845/.

World Health Organization. 2020. *Depression.* https://www.who.int/news-room/fact-sheets/detail/depression

Koskie, B. K. *Depression: Facts, Statistics, and You.* Healthline.com. June 3, 2020. https://www.healthline.com/health/depression/facts-statistics-infographic.

Schrodt, P. *Here's how much it costs to get an A-list celebrity to show up at your party.* BUSINESS INSIDER. August 7, 2016. https://www.google.com/amp/s/www.businessinsider.com/booking-celebrities-at-parties-2016-8%3famp

Tyko, K. McDonald's popular Travis Scott Meal now available for $6 with fast-food chain's mobile app through Oct. 4. USA TODAY. September 22, 2020.

https://www.goodmorningamerica.com/amp/food/story/rapper-travis-scott-mcdonalds-meal-1st-celebrity-collaboration-72876178

Principle #3

Ortner, N. O. *A Short Lesson on Gratitude.* The Tapping Solution. https://www.thetappingsolution.com/blog/short-lesson-gratitude/

WIKIPEDIA. 2020. *Maslow's hierarchy of needs.* https://en.m.wikipedia.org/wiki/Maslow%27s_hierarchy_of_needs

Frankl, V. E. (2006). *Man's Search for Meaning.* Beacon Press.

Lieberman, D. (2014). *The Story of the Human Body: Evolution, Health, and*

Disease. Vintage.

Principle #4

Burnell, C. B. *A little history of reading: How the first books came to be.* BookTrust. December 3, 2019. https://www.booktrust.org.uk/news-and-features/features/2019/december/a-little-history-of-reading-how-the-first-books-came-to-be/

Morgan, K. M. *What Are the Benefits of Attending Seminars?* https://education.seattlepi.com/benefits-attending-seminars-1929.html.

Government of South Australia. 2020. *The Risks of Poor Nutrition.*

World Health Organization. 2020. *Global Strategy on Diet, Physical Activity and Health: Diet, nutrition and the prevention of chronic diseases.* https://www.who.int/dietphysicalactivity/publications/trs916/summary/en/.

Ryan T. Hurt, MD, PhD, Christopher Kulisek, MD, and Stephen A. McClave, MD. 2010. *The Obesity Epidemic: Challenges, Health Initiatives, and Implications for Gastroenterologists.* NCBI. https://www.ncbi.nlm.nih.gov/pmc/articles/PMC3033553/.

Centers for Disease Control and Prevention. *Overweight & Obesity.* June 29, 2020. https://www.cdc.gov/obesity/data/adult.html.

Centers for Disease Control and Prevention. Jan 2020. *LDL and HDL Cholesterol: "Bad" and "Good" Cholesterol.*

Girard, S. E. *The Body's Fuel Sources.* Human Kinetics. https://us.humankinetics.com/blogs/excerpt/the-bodys-fuel-sources.

Nordqvist, J. N. *How much sugar is in your food and drink?* MedicalNewsToday. February 14, 2018. https://www.medicalnewstoday.com/articles/262978#what-is-sugar.

Anon. *Quick Tips: Adding Fruits and Vegetables to Your Diet.* HealthLinkBC. August 22, 2019. https://www.healthlinkbc.ca/health-topics/ud3719.

Anon. *Fish and Omega-3 Fatty Acids.* Heart.org. March 23, 2017. https://www.heart.org/en/healthy-living/healthy-eating/eat-smart/fats/fish-and-omega-3-fatty-acids.

Brazier, Y. B. *How much salt should a person eat?* MedicalNewsToday. July

28, 2017. https://www.medicalnewstoday.com/articles/146677#uses

Principle #5

How Socializing Can Keep Your Brain Healthy. BRAINCHECK. January 10, 2018. https://braincheck.com/blog/how-socializing-keeps-brain-healthy.

Anon. *The Importance of Friendship: A story about a little boy and his hands and feet.* KABBALAH. http://www.kabbalah.info/eng/content/view/frame/59460?/eng/content/view/full/59460&main.

Blue, A. B. *Poor Social Skills May Be Harmful to Mental and Physical Health.* The University of Arizona. Nov. 6, 2017. https://news.arizona.edu/story/poor-social-skills-may-be-harmful-mental-and-physical-health.

Baum, I. B. *How Your Body Can React To Chronic Isolation.* Bustle. November 29, 2016. https://www.bustle.com/articles/196816-11-things-that-can-happen-to-your-mind-body-if-you-dont-socialize-for-a.

Doyle, A. D. *Important Teamwork Skills That Employers Value.* The balancecareer. November 24, 2019. https://www.thebalancecareers.com/list-of-teamwork-skills-2063773.

The Oracles. *12 tips from successful execs on how to stop negative people from getting in your way.* BUSINESS INSIDER. December 30, 2017. https://www.google.com/amp/s/www.businessinsider.com/12-execs-share-how-to-stop-negative-people-from-getting-in-your-way-2017-12%3famp

Principle #6

William L. Hosch. *Steve Wozniak.* Britannica. https://www.britannica.com/biography/Stephen-Gary-Wozniak.

Beattie, A. B. *Steve Jobs and the Apple Story: The legacy and lessons of Apple's co-founder.* Investopedia. March 14, 2020. https://www.investopedia.com/articles/fundamental-analysis/12/steve-jobs-apple-story.asp.

Eds. *Wright Brothers.* June 6, 2019. https://www.google.com/amp/s/www.history.com/.amp/topics/inventions/wright-brothers.

Zetlin, M. Z. *Blockbuster Could Have Bought Netflix for $50 Million, but the CEO Thought It Was a Joke.* Inc. September 20, 2019. https://www.inc.com/mindazetlin/netflix-blockbuster-meeting-marc-randolph-reed-hastings-john-antioco.html.

James Manyika, Michael Chui, Jacques Bughin, Richard Dobbs, Peter Bisson, and Alex Marrs. *Disruptive technologies: Advances that will transform life, business, and the global economy.* McKinsey Global Institute. May 1, 2013. https://www.mckinsey.com/business-functions/mckinsey-digital/our-insights/disruptive-technologies.

Kenton, W. K. *Groupthink.* Investopedia. August 24, 2020. https://www.investopedia.com/terms/g/groupthink.asp.

Principle #7

Williams, C. W. *Five ways science can improve your focus.* BBC. 25th September 2017. https://www.bbc.com/worklife/article/20170925-the-surprising-tricks-to-help-you-focus-at-work.

ScienceDirect. *Effects of breaks on regaining vitality at work: An empirical comparison of 'conventional' and 'smart phone' breaks.* April 2016. https://www.sciencedirect.com/science/article/abs/pii/S0747563215302703.

Boss, J. B. *5 Reasons Why Goal Setting Will Improve Your Focus.* Forbes. January 19, 2017. https://www.google.com/amp/s/www.forbes.com/sites/jeffboss/2017/01/19/5-reasons-why-goal-setting-will-improve-your-focus/amp/

James, G. J. *What Goal-Setting Does to Your Brain and Why It's Spectacularly Effective.* Inc. October 23, 2019. https://www.inc.com/geoffrey-james/what-goal-setting-does-to-your-brain-why-its-spectacularly-effective.html

Sáez, F. S. *Resting Properly, Key to Your Productivity.* https://facilethings.com/blog/en/rest

Habits: How They Form And How To Break Them. NPR.org. March 5, 2012. https://www.npr.org/2012/03/05/147192599/habits-how-they-form-and-how-to-break-themhttps://www.investopedia.com/terms/g/groupthink.asp

Principle #8

Susan M. Heathfield. *How to Take Responsibility for Your Life: When You Take

Responsibility for Your Life, You Achieve Your Dreams. The balancecareer. January 5, 2020. https://www.thebalancecareers.com/how-to-take-responsibility-for-your-life-1919214#:~:text=The%20most%20important%20aspect%20of,you%20made%20and%20are%20making.

Possing, S. P. *How to be responsible.* wikiHow. September 29, 2020. https://www.wikihow.com/Be-Responsible?amp=1

45 Famous Failures Who Became Successful People. https://www.develop-goodhabits.com/successful-people-failed/

Ducharme, J. D. *The Sunk Cost Fallacy Is Ruining Your Decisions. Here's How.* TIME. July 26, 2018. https://www.google.com/amp/s/time.com/5347133/sunk-cost-fallacy-decisions/%3famp=true

Derrick, J. D. *Remember When Yahoo Turned Down $1 Million To Buy Google?* Yahoo! Finance. July 25, 2016. https://www.google.com/amp/s/finance.yahoo.com/amphtml/news/remember-yahoo-turned-down-1-132805083.html

Solomon, B. S. *How Jerry Yang Killed Yahoo, By Saving It.* Forbes. Jul 25, 2016. https://www.forbes.com/sites/briansolomon/2016/07/25/yahoo-verizon-sold-alibaba-jerry-yang/amp/

Overconfidence Bias – You Are Not As Smart As You Think. Productive Club. https://productiveclub.com/overconfidence-bias/

Principle #9

Patrick R. Heck. *65% of Americans believe they are above average in intelligence: Results of two nationally representative surveys.* NCBI. https://www.ncbi.nlm.nih.gov/pmc/articles/PMC6029792/

Penn Today. *What factors predict success? New research from Angela Duckworth and colleagues finds that characteristics beyond intelligence influence long-term achievement.* https://penntoday.upenn.edu/news/Penn-Angela-Duckworth-looks-beyond-grit-predict-success

Duckworth, Angela L., Peterson, Christopher, Matthews, Michael D., Kelly, Dennis R. *Grit: Perseverance and passion for long-term goals.* APA PsycNet. Jun 2007. https://psycnet.apa.org/buy/2007-07951-009.

Lebowitz, S. L. *Why Your IQ May Have More Influence on Your Success*

Than You Think: You could more accurately predict a job candidate's future performance with a holistic approach that measures IQ and social skills. Inc. Oct 9, 2017. https://www.inc.com/business-insider/why-iq-big-factor-future-success-job-performance-according-science-research.html

Acharya, M. *11-year-old Indian origin student Kashmea Wahi beats Albert Einstein's IQ Score.*

Taylor, N. R. *Stephen Hawking Biography (1942-2018).* SPACE.com. 2018. https://www.google.com/amp/s/www.space.com/amp/15923-stephen-hawking.html

National Library of Medicine (NIH). *The nature of adolescent competencies predicted by preschool delay of gratification.* W Mischel et al. J Pers Soc Psychol. 1988 Apr. https://pubmed.ncbi.nlm.nih.gov/3367285/

National Library of Medicine. *Delay of gratification in children.* W Mischel et al. Science. 1989. https://pubmed.ncbi.nlm.nih.gov/2658056/

Predicting Adolescent Cognitive and Self-Regulatory Competencies From Preschool Delay of Gratification: Identifying Diagnostic Conditions. Research Gate. November 1990.

https://www.researchgate.net/publication/232585605_Predicting_Adolescent_Cognitive_and_SelfRegulatory_Competencies_From_Preschool_Delay_of_Gratification_Identifying_Diagnostic_Conditions.

www.ingramcontent.com/pod-product-compliance
Lightning Source LLC
Chambersburg PA
CBHW051257250726
48656CB00004B/1337